SpringerBriefs in Public Health

SpringerBriefs in Public Health present concise summaries of cutting-edge research and practical applications from across the entire field of public health, with contributions from medicine, bioethics, health economics, public policy, biostatistics, and sociology.

The focus of the series is to highlight current topics in public health of interest to a global audience, including health care policy; social determinants of health; health issues in developing countries; new research methods; chronic and infectious disease epidemics; and innovative health interventions.

Featuring compact volumes of 55 to 125 pages, the series covers a range of content from professional to academic. Possible volumes in the series may consist of timely reports of state-of-the art analytical techniques, reports from the field, snapshots of hot and/or emerging topics, literature reviews, and in-depth case studies. Both solicited and unsolicited manuscripts are considered for publication in this series.

Briefs are published as part of Springer's eBook collection, with millions of users worldwide. In addition, Briefs are available for individual print and electronic purchase.

Briefs are characterized by fast, global electronic dissemination, standard publishing contracts, easy-to-use manuscript preparation and formatting guidelines, and expedited production schedules. We aim for publication 8–12 weeks after acceptance.

Töres Theorell

Underuse of Applied Science in Changing Societies

Trust in Applied Science Among Lay People

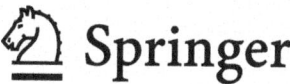 Springer

Töres Theorell
Global Health
Karolinska Institutet
Stockholm, Sweden

ISSN 2192-3698   ISSN 2192-3701   (electronic)
SpringerBriefs in Public Health
ISBN 978-3-031-96390-2   ISBN 978-3-031-96391-9   (eBook)
https://doi.org/10.1007/978-3-031-96391-9

This Springer imprint is published by the registered company Springer Nature Switzerland AG
The registered company address is: Gewerbestrasse 11, 6330 Cham, Switzerland

If disposing of this product, please recycle the paper.

Preface

There are several indications that findings from applied science are underutilized by modern societies. Applied science is intended to help when we are about to make decisions about difficult problems. For instance, we might need statistical computations about ways of building bridges. How many years is it likely that the bridge will remain useful without falling apart? And if we want an even more sustainable bridge, how much more will it cost according to statistics based upon experiences from other kinds of bridge building? Health care planning also utilizes statistics. Decision making based upon applied science could be regarded as the modern way of solving conflicts. If we do not use applied science in society's decision making we are wasting a lot of money. So, what are the reasons for the neglect of not using applied science?

When we are discussing the role of applied science in society it is important for us to know *who they are, those who produce the findings!* Perhaps assertiveness (too much or too little?) in the researchers themselves could be one factor that we should discuss when we try to understand the role of applied science. There are many parties involved in producing and listening to applied science—from scientists and research students to those who produce books and articles, journalists who write about the results, and politicians and administrators who choose or do not choose to listen to what the scientific results tell us. We cannot single out one of them. Let me start with an egocentric and myopic view of myself. This is of course an important background for my choice of examples as well as for my way of discussing and choosing topics for this book. And I have had many experiences of applied science myself— even if these experiences are limited they will tell something about applied science in general.

I am just pretending to be a researcher is a sentence that I have carried with me throughout my career as a researcher, initially in clinical research while I was a clinically active physician and then as a full-time researcher during several decades. My mantra tells me that I am not really a researcher, I am just moving around in the vicinity of science. That feeling is still a dominating one. This is despite the fact that I am retired after having served as a professor with the main task of doing research and in addition having been recorded (according to Research Gate 2022) as main author or co-author of more than 700 scientific publications, 480 of which are available in the international database Medline/PubMed. I have also supervised the production of 47 doctoral theses.

According to Research Gate on the 20th of February 2022, there were 42,525 quotations of studies that I have been part of. All of that has no importance for my self-image as a just an almost scientist, I do not feel like a real researcher. This could be both a strength and a weakness.

My biochemist father is behind my mantra. He knew all the technical aspects of how to do basic research and he did not consider public health or epidemiological research to be real research. The feeling of not being a "real scientist" has been with me all the time. My father who was otherwise a considerate and reasonable person was clear in his distancing from "science depending on statistics." Only late in his life did he accept that there could be a causal relationship between tobacco smoking and lung cancer.

In addition, it was typical for a nature scientist in his era to be a developmental optimist—science will always find solutions when new problems arise in the world. And it is probably true that his field basic science has been more popular than the field applied science that I have spent my life in.

A major difference between my father's research era and my own was the low level of formalities in his world. To some extent this mirrors a more relaxed time. But it is also related to the strong position that basic science had at the time and to the fact that science on the whole was occupying a smaller group of researchers and a much more informal approach was acceptable. He used to tell us a story about how he "applied" for research money on one particular occasion. He needed to expand his laboratory building and went up to one of Sweden's most wealthy men at the time, Jakob Wallenberg, who asked: Why would I put money into this? Theorell's not very specified answer was: *A shoemaker uses a form when he produces a shoe. This is approximately what we do in biochemical research—we find out how life is constructed so that people get useful forms for constructing a good society.* He received his money. However, he was a very good storyteller, so he probably improved the real story substantially. It may not have been that easy! It should be kept in mind that Hugo Theorell's name was in high regard both nationally and internationally (Rockefeller foundation for instance), and that still makes a difference today, in the same way as it did during his time. But compared to formalities required to obtain research grants today, it was indeed simpler.

That Sweden avoided participation in the two world wars was an important factor in the Swedish international position during the late 1940s until the 1980s. It was possible to build a welfare state with emphasis on equality, arts, and science. My father had advantage in this situation, and so did I in the beginning of my career—Sweden had allocated resources to work environment and public health research, my own areas. However, during the later part of my career I felt that Sweden's favorable position had been weakened. Other countries had reached our level or even passed it. We should remember that Nobel prizes in natural science (physics, chemistry, and medicine/physiology) are almost exclusively devoted to basic science and not to applied science which is the main theme of this book. That probably also explains why applied science has less assertiveness than basic science. This could be one of the many explanations for underutilization of applied science.

Coming back to my somewhat derogatory statements about my own research as not "real" research: The crucial discussion is about basic versus applied research. My father was doing biochemical basic research while I have mainly been doing applied research associated directly with clinical and epidemiological public health questions. There is a floating border between the two. In my imagination while I was a child, basic research should be about chemistry, physics, mathematics, biology, and new discoveries in nature. But the most important differentiation is probably that basic research is about exploring the unknown. This means doing basic research for its own sake, without glancing at immediate utility. This is the charming aspect of basic science, and the corresponding way of thinking has influenced my own attitude to my research in a positive way—despite that I have not been doing basic research. Basic science is at its best when it does not have to constantly prove utility. The most important groundbreaking discoveries have been made by scientists whose goal was to discover the unknown, not to be immediately useful to society. This means that playing should be an important component and that there has to be allowance for the fact that most of the scientific activities do not lead to great discoveries. One paradox is that mistakes could lead to important discovery. One of the most well-known examples is Fleming's discovery of penicillin. Fleming one day left his laboratory for summer vacation and by accident left bacteria plates. When he came back the bacteria had been growing excessively, but in places where there was penicillin there was no growth—a discovery of historical magnitude.

The penicillin example, of course, does not mean that mistakes are recommended in science. But society must show tolerance for the need for playing and trial and error in research. It should also be pointed out that Fleming's discovery in bacteriology may not have been developed into such a success had he not collaborated with another discipline, biochemistry. Florey and Chain, the two biochemists that he collaborated with, had great importance and shared the Nobel Prize with Fleming. Accordingly, a major reason why Fleming's mistake and discovery of penicillin became a success was that his science was embedded in a professional environment which allows playing and mistakes. There is less tolerance for playing and mistakes in applied science which is closer to politics and societal administration. This also means that politicians may suddenly decide that financial support to some sector of applied science should be withdrawn—for ideological reasons. Thus, applied science is more vulnerable to political currents in society than basic science is.

Laypeople whose knowledge about research is limited may feel fascination with unexpected discoveries in basic science, such as new planetary systems, previously unknown fish species, new principles in physics which can be applied in communication, discoveries of techniques for building violins in the eighteenth century, methods for studying age of archaeological objects, or new principles for treating or preventing dementia. Applied science may be less spectacular but is nevertheless extremely important for our survival. Examples of what applied science can help us with are to evaluate effects of new treatments in medicine, test sustainability of materials for house building, explore health effects of bad work organization, examine effects of different forms of societal efforts to limit use of alcohol, tobacco, and mobile phones, and find out in epidemiological studies about material and social conditions in different parts of the population. That may not be so spectacular from the point of view of citizens in general as discoveries in basic science. But the evaluation of effects of a newly discovered pharmacological agent, for instance, is quite complicated and requires obedience to the statistical methods and ethical principles. Otherwise, laypeople cannot trust that the new product has beneficial effects and that it is not harmful.

Another dividing line: There is clearly also a difference between humanistic and natural sciences regarding the average citizen's trust in different kinds of research. This is mirrored in annual assessments of trust in different kinds of societal institutions in Sweden (SOM-rapport 2021:18, Vetenskapen i Samhället). There is a pronounced difference between medical science on one hand (from 2002 to 2020 between 64% and 88% of the population reported good or fairly good trust in medical science) and societal science on the other hand (with corresponding percentages 37% to 54%). There were no obvious time trends; trust in those kinds of sciences does not seem to vane or grow markedly. My own field stress research has components of both medical and societal research. Sometimes I have been more societal and sometimes more medical. If we assume that people's trust in my kind of research is between that of medical/natural science (year average 77%) and societal science (49%), it means that on average 63% feel trust in "my" research. That may sound OK, but it means that 37% of people reading articles about it in newspapers or social media are likely to distrust it. When I report strictly medical results (for instance, levels of stress hormones in defined situations) there may only be 23% who distrust me but when I report epidemiological findings from a scientific exploration of psychosocial factors at work in relation to some illness risk, 51% may distrust me. During later years, governmental commissions on science have emphasized the importance of a strong development of natural, medical, and technical science, more or less at the expense of humanistic and societal science. I feel tempted to conclude that these commissions have not realized that the introduction into a changing society of discoveries in the "hard" sciences requires deep, up-to-date knowledge in humanistic and societal science.

Although I merely look at myself as a guest in science I have still experienced a lot as a scholar during five decades. Perhaps my feeling of being a bystander has been a strength since I have been able to use a bystander perspective in difficult situations. Or perhaps it was a weakness because it may have decreased my engagement?

But my main question arising from my experiences and from the division between basic and applied research that arose for family reasons very early in my career has grown strongly during my years as a researcher:

Why is society not listening seriously to applied research? As I have argued the problem of mistrust is less for basic research than it is for applied research. Therefore, I will focus on applied research in this book and discuss the problems from many points of view, from the production and producer side, from society perspectives, and from the perspective of stakeholders and decision makers. Most of the more detailed examples that I use are from my own experiences. However, I believe that they represent experiences from applied research in general.

The main question in this book is presently of dramatic importance in the world since the scientific leading country's political leaders are questioning the usefulness of applied science and even threaten the whole financial federal system that has supported it for many decades. Therefore, we have to describe and analyze our basic understanding of how applied science works and what its strengths and weaknesses are. And why its position is not as strong as it should be.

Stockholm, Sweden   Töres Theorell

Reference

SOM-rapport. (2021). *Vetenskapen i Samhället (Science in Society)*. SOM-report 2021:18. Gothenburg University.

Contents

About the Author

Töres Theorell, PhD, MD retired professor of psychosocial medicine at the Karolinska Institutet in Stockholm, Sweden, was born in 1942, became a licensed physician at the Karolinska Institutet in Stockholm in 1967, and defended his PhD thesis in 1971. He worked in clinical medicine (internal medicine and cardiology) and was appointed professor of health care research and from 1995 professor of psychosocial medicine at the Karolinska Institutet. After retirement he has been a scientific consultant at the Department of Psychology at the University of Stockholm and also a lecturer at the Royal College of Music in Stockholm. Theorell is author/co-author of 486 articles available in Medline. His bibliometric D-index is 92. He has supervised 47 doctoral students. He is a member of the Academia Europaea. His research has been in epidemiological and physiological aspects of cardiovascular disease and depression as in intervention research.

Introduction: Why Do People Not Listen?

A recent dramatic example illustrates that even high-status people may mistrust the results produced by applied science. The newly elected president of the United States of America, Donald Trump, gave an interview (Cleetus, 2025) where he was asked the question, "But what happens now when you have decided to leave the Paris Treaty and to allow increased carbon dioxide production? Scientists now say in unison that the carbon dioxide increase is causing climate change." His response: "No, I do not think the scientists know that." This is one of the most negative statements I know about an advanced concerted effort in applied science. Mr. Trump had no argument supporting this statement, but his negative attitude has had a disastrous effect on the world's work on the climate change problem.

Democracy has been threatened in many countries in the free world. The same is true of applied science. It could be argued that in a world situation where increasing numbers of people distrust politicians, applied science might be the sector people should turn to for advice. After all, applied science has arisen and developed due to the need for relevant fact-based knowledge for decisions in our societies. Quite to the contrary, knowledge from applied science has been utilized to a decreasing extent (Kuhlmann et al., 2022). In the ideal world, from the scientist's wishful point of view, scientific policy advice is expected to fulfill the double function of pushing evidence-based policymaking while improving the legitimacy of political decisions (Bogumil & Jann, 2020). Another way of saying it is that scientific policy advice aims to produce knowledge that is not only "factually correct and resilient," but also politically useful (Weingart & Lentsch, 2008).

The interplay between applied science and politics can be described according to contrasting theoretical models. There is a *decisionist* model wherein political-administrative actors are conceived as dominating the process and making use of experts' knowledge, which is assumed to be without bias. In the other extreme, according to the *technocratic* model, scientific expertise is assumed to have superiority in every problem-solving situation. Thus, the scientists are supposed to be able to find solutions to all problems, which reduces the role of administrators and

T. Theorell, *Underuse of Applied Science in Changing Societies*, SpringerBriefs in Public Health, https://doi.org/10.1007/978-3-031-96391-9_1

politicians to executors of directives from the scientists (Martinsen & Rehfeld, 2006). Habermas described a more realistic *pragmatic* model (Aboulafia et al., 2002). According to that model, political-administrative decisions are seen as results of an iterative process between actors, either involved in scientific policy advice or in decision-making, as well as a translation process between science and politics.

One of the problems is that the number of results being produced in applied science has been increasing, and these results often diverge. In this situation, laymen tend to select the research results that confirm their ideas. They do this instead of taking advice from groups of scientists who are familiar with the discussion considering the pros and cons. If politicians would rather "cherry pick" the results they want to see, one could ask whether it is meaningful to expect politicians to make use of results from applied science. If society is increasingly less willing to listen, the politicians may start to question why they should allocate money to applied science.

Figure 1 provides an overview of trust and distrust back and forth between researchers, as well as between researchers and the surrounding society. Distrust between researchers contributes to distrust between applied science (researchers) and society. When there is distrust between applied science and society, it affects the research community itself. The researchers could join forces and help each other, or they could react more egotistically, trying to save their positions. Distrust and trust in science arises from interactions between society and researchers.

What explanations can we find for the contemporary lack of interest and trust in applied science? There seem to be many different layers of explanations. The goal of this book is to go through the most important ones, some of which lie in the surrounding societies and some of which lie in the scientific society itself, including how new generations of scientists are educated and how they obey the rules of scientific activity. There has always been quarreling and distrust within the scientific community itself. A letter (quoted in Clark, 1985) from a famous basic scientist, Ernst Boris Chain, one of the three Nobel Prize recipients in 1945 for penicillin, reveals his deep feeling of distrust in researchers in general:

> The scientist looking for ultimate guidance in questions of moral responsibility would do well to recognize the limitations and fallacies in this respect of the scientific approach, to abandon the status of intellectual superiority with which he has vested, often against his wish, by wide circles in the lay public, largely as a result of the concepts of nineteenth-century scientific philosophy, and to turn, or return, to the fundamental and lasting values

Fig. 1 Trust and distrust between researchers, and between researchers and society (Credit: Annika Röhl, 2025)

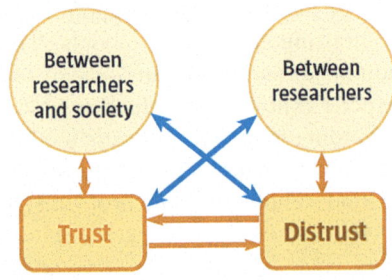

of the code of ethical behavior forming part of the divine message which man was uniquely privileged to receive through the intermediation of a few chosen individuals.

Chain's philosophy was grounded in his Jewish upbringing, but his message is not propaganda for any religion but rather a fundamental belief that scientific activity must be founded in ethical norms and moral responsibility. This deep conviction has influenced many of the most famous scientists who have been ready to defend the truth. In parts of this book, I shall describe some tools with which applied science tries to formalize moral responsibility and fight against faked results, amplifications, premature presentation of results, and other dishonest expressions, which all in the end threaten the credibility of science in the eyes of lay people.

Ernst Chain's statement also illustrates the difference between basic and applied science. He talks about those in basic science as "...a few chosen individuals." Basic science is indeed about the discovery of previously unknown conditions. This requires unusual creativity, which is an unusual quality. His point is that those individuals have great responsibility and must "turn, or return, to the fundamental and lasting values of the code of ethical behavior forming part of the divine message..." Although applied science does not require this unique degree of creativity, those in the field of applied science have to follow the same high ethical standards as those in basic science.

This book uses Sweden, a small European country with old and strong democratic and scientific traditions, as an empirical example. One special feature of Sweden is that it did not participate in the First and Second World Wars. This is one of the reasons scientific production in our country did not experience a sudden halt. In some ways, Sweden had a scientific advantage in comparison to other countries immediately after WWII. Politicians in Sweden realized that rapid scientific development was an asset. The most important international research fund, the Rockefeller Foundation, has awarded significant funds to Swedish researchers (see p 73, Huldt et al., 2013). In light of this, Sweden could be seen as a country with an unbroken development of applied science and is thus of special interest in efforts to describe a spontaneous development essentially uninterrupted by disasters. What follows is a discussion of how the volume of applied science production increased after the Second World War in Sweden and how this development is paralleled by decreasing trust in the products it has generated.

Basic science had a stronger position 100 years ago. Chapin expressed gratitude for major discoveries in the US that advanced efforts to fight against pandemics and improve public health (Chapin, 1927).

My research fields in applied science, including *psychosocial medicine* and *culture and health,* have each had relatively low status, although both topics have substantial potential in society. The reasons are probably different in each case. Regarding psychosomatic medicine, it is often hard for laymen and experts in other fields to accept that mental processes could contribute to pathology in bodily organs, although there is massive proof that this is indeed the case. With regard to culture and health, the problem is that most politicians are ready to say favorable things about culture, but most of them are not ready to finance it. An underlying problem may be the wide acceptance that cultural activities can be energizing for both individuals and societies, but from the politician's point of view, it is often hard to know in which direction this energy will take the population—either for or against that politician. A brutal illustration of one society's unwillingness to accept cultural expressions is seen under the rule of the Taliban, which prohibits most kinds of cultural activities in Afghanistan (ABC News, 2021). A politician's fear of uncontrollable political movements stimulated by cultural activities is not the lone possible explanation for prohibition of culture in Afghanistan. Strong religious conviction among the leaders is, of course, the official reason, but the real reason is very likely to be the reason behind the strong force with which the prohibition is driven.

One important contemporary discussion (Knaggård, 2009) relates to our society's handling of scientific data coming from climate change research. This field relies on scientific and technological studies. As expected, the societal impact of the research results depends on the interaction between scientists and society. It was shown that scientific uncertainty is one of many factors that affect political decisions. Policymakers had many ways of making decisions when scientific results were unclear. Reframing the issue, making uncertainties irrelevant, demanding the precautionary principle (demanding more research), and awaiting future recommendations from the scientists were the most common principles used. Despite the reality that scientists have been important in the formulation of climate change as a *societal problem*, the result has been that scientists have had a very small real influence on the formulation of *climate policy*.

Another example illustrating the underutilization of applied science in Sweden is their handling of primary health care. The system employs primary care physicians in the public sector, as has been the case with the whole health care sector, including hospital care. In recent years, several political parties have been pushing for privatization, particularly for the primary care sector. In Stockholm, Sweden's capital city, drastic changes have taken place. One important consequence is that it has become much more difficult to organize public health initiatives. Regional authorities have lost influence over where to establish new privatized primary healthcare centers. As a result, areas with strong public health outcomes have a much higher density of primary healthcare centers compared to regions with poor public health, and the costs for primary healthcare have increased substantially (Mosquera et al., 2021). In addition, the performance of ambulatory care under sensitive conditions (cases in which adequate handled by primary care could prevent hospitalization) was worse in privatized centers. All of these consequences had been predicted with warnings issued by scientists. The politicians chose not to listen to the research predicting adverse consequences.

Public health promotion has become more challenging as health care districts lose defined geographic boundaries, leading to varied disease prevalence across regions. This erodes health care staff's localized knowledge, rendering area-specific health promotion less effective.

Developments parallel to the healthcare situation have taken place in the education system. Politicians in power have listened more to their political ideology than to the insights of applied research. The results have been disappointing. Primary healthcare has become dysfunctional, and the Swedish school system, which occupied an top position internationally in educational achievements according to PISA (Programme for International Student Assessment), has had a declining position for several years (OECD, 2019). However, the politicians in the largest city-county, Stockholm, continued to stimulate privatization along with other changes, resulting in adverse effects despite repeated OECD (Organization for Economic Cooperation and Development) warnings to Swedish politicians. Thus, political ideology turned out to be more relevant than results from applied research.

There are threats to applied science coming from external sources—as politicians and higher administration officials increasingly disregard applied science—but also from inside. Researchers reporting results dishonestly or in exaggerated ways and researchers who avoid results that do not confirm their hypotheses are eroding the trust in applied science. The problem of mistrust has many facets, and this book shall discuss some of them. When discussing the multifaceted reasons behind society's relatively small interest in applied science, a general overview is provided, which is illustrated in Fig. 2. There is a flow between the groups that produce applied science results as well as between them and all the groups in society that use (or do not use) their results. Financial conditions are decisive, and society determines those, but financial decisions depend upon how useful the results are considered to be for administration and policy making.

Chapter "Introduction: Why Do People Not Listen?" introduces the reasons behind society's failure to heed scientific evidence, setting the stage for the book's analysis of applied science's challenges.

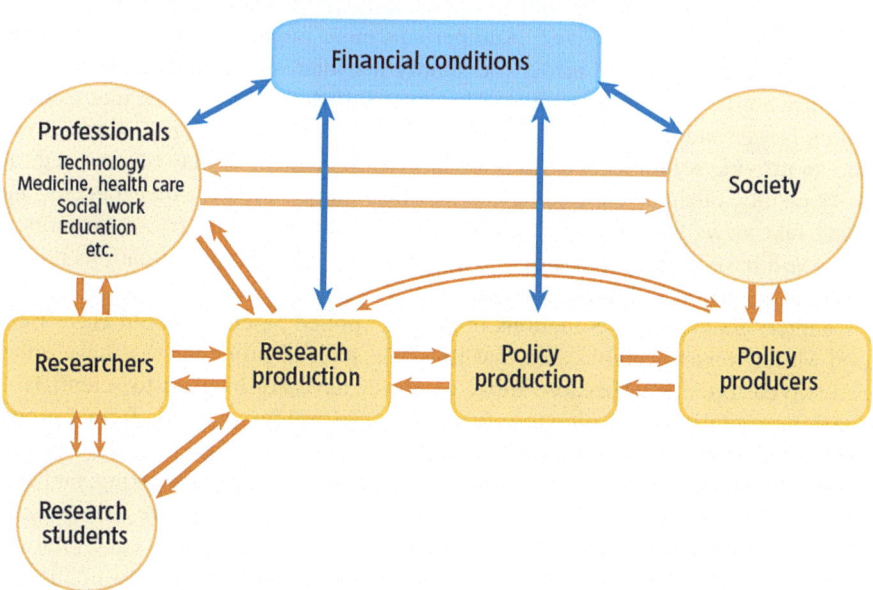

Fig. 2 Production and acceptance of applied research (Credit: Annika Röhl, 2025)

Chapter "Production and Producers," posits that there are material conditions, such as financial support, that influence how many collaborators can be employed as well as how skillful these collaborators are and how many "muscles" applied science will have.

Chapter "Research Students," asserts that researchers recruited for applied science have great importance. Their way of thinking is influenced by their reasons for entering the field and the attitudes they face in society and the research community. If there is general distrust between society and applied research, this is likely to reduce the recruitment of those talented in research.

Chapter "How Does Applied Science Operate?" argues that the research community itself is important for credibility. I shall try to describe one big undertaking that I was involved in myself. This shows how a large group of researchers in several countries made a joint effort to find methods for describing psychosocial work environments and how these relate to work-related illness risks. This counters common beliefs that applied research results arise in the heads of researchers, ending up as useless books on bookshelves, representing just one kind of pressure group in society. It also illustrates that diversity in opinion is a necessary ingredient in scientific production. Intense competition between researchers can increase engagement and tempo, but also increases the risk of faking and dishonest reporting of results.

Chapter "Communication With Society," presents the community surrounding applied science as a factor that merits discussion. To what extent do lay people have trust in science? Are people self-centered when they try to understand results from applied science, therefore dismissing collective aspects? A related question is: "To what extent do people accept results that point to solutions which are not beneficial for them as individuals in the short term, even though the solutions may be preferable in a long-term perspective?" And perhaps more important than anything else: In some countries, those in power are simply not interested in providing the solutions that are best for most people. The most selfish ones are more interested in gaining power and money for themselves. For them, applied science is an activity that can provide solutions benefiting themselves. For them, it may be important to falsify results, misinterpret findings so that they can be used for their benefit, and spread fake news to large numbers of people. Politicians who try to use correct results will have the tough task of convincing others and creating situations that do not allow distortion and faking of data.

Chapter "Examples of Situations in Which Applied Science Should Have Been Used More," reviews eight cases that illustrate societal problems that have either been solved too slowly because those in power have not listened to scientists or expect their solution to develop too slowly into a diffuse future. In the former group, we find the closing of an airport, pollution of waste products resulting in death and serious illness in the population, dangers associated with tobacco smoking, and dangers of bad psychosocial work environments. In the latter group, we find possible public health effects of wind turbines, simplistic recommendations of easy solutions of shyness in children, hasty, careless privatization of health care, and finally, the solution of the world's climate crisis due to carbon dioxide pollution.

Chapter "Solutions," will discuss what the research community can do to improve the situation. A primary key is to expand the knowledge among lay people regarding what applied science can do and how it works. That should start primarily in the school system. If children learn more about how science works, they will be more likely to listen to arguments from applied science.

Chapter "Conclusions," summarizes the main themes. Perhaps the most important conclusion is that we need to increase knowledge about what applied research is and how it works..

Figure 2 (in this chapter) shows the complex relationships between the different actors in the production of applied research. Some professionals give input to the researchers—what are the most important areas that you should pay attention to in your research? This is represented by the arrows between these groups. The professionals influence the researchers and vice versa. In this book, we shall discuss several examples. One of the positive examples is the process illustrating how obstetric nurses start wondering whether the practice of dripping silver nitrate into the eyes of newborn babies should be continued. The routine of doing so was created before the antibiotic era, when a gonorrhea infection in the genitalia of the mother could infect the eyes of the babies and make them blind. However, the obstetric nurses suspected that this was not necessary because we now have modern antibiotics that could prevent blindness in babies. And the benefits of silver nitrate drops should be weighed against the adverse effects arising from the contact between the baby and mother because the baby shuts the nitrate-aching eyes for the first days. So applied research in that case was about objectively recording for how long the eyes were shut and what that could mean for the child's development. This research resulted in the abandonment of the silver nitrate drops routine. There are other positive examples in the book.

Figure 2 also illustrates the back-and-forth relationships between researchers and their research students. We will discuss the following relationships. Who is recruited to applied research and how is the relationship between these groups functioning? Professionals, researchers, and research students are the central forces in research production. The directions for research production are determined by policy production and by financial conditions that vary from period to period and from area to area.

References

ABC News. (2021, August). *Taliban pose threat to Afghan cultural heritage as they sweep back into power - By Conor Finnegan.*

Aboulafia, M., Bookman, M., & Kemp, C. (2002). Habermas and pragmatism. In M. Aboulafia, M. Bookman, & C. Kemp (Eds.), *Habermas and pragmatism. Philosophy reviews.* Routledge.

Bogumil, J., & Jann, W. (2020, June 16). *Verwaltung und Verwaltungswissenschaft in Deutschland.* Springer Fachmedien Wiesbaden. isbn:9783658284084.

Chapin, C. V. (1927). Science and public health. *American Journal of Public Health, 17,* 1109–1116.

Clark, R. W. (1985). *The life of Ernst Chain. Penicillin and beyond.* Weidenfeld and Nicolson.

Cleetus, R. (2025, January). *President Trump ignores science, makes disgraceful statement to withdraw US from Paris Agreement. Union of concerned scientists.*

Huldt, I., Normark, D., & Norrving, B. (2013). *Från läkarskola till medicinskt universitet. Karolinska Institutets ledning 1953-2012 (From physician school to medical university. The management of the Karolinska Institutet 1953-2012).* Karolinska Institutet University Press. isbn:9789185565634.

Knaggård, Å. (2009). *Vetenskaplig osäkerhet i policyprocessen. En studie av svensk klimatpolitik (Scientific uncertainty in the policy process. A study of Swedish climate politics).* Doctoral thesis. Statsvetenskapliga institutionen (Department of Political Science), Lund University.

Kuhlmann, S., Franzke, J., & Dumas, B. P. (2022). Technocratic decision-making in times of crisis? The use of data for scientific policy advice in Germany's COVID-19 management. *Public Organization Review, 22*(2), 269–289. https://doi.org/10.1007/s11115-022-00635-8. PMCID: PMC9185129.

Martinsen, R., & Rehfeld, D. (2006). Von der Aufklärung über Defizite zur reflexiven Aufklärung? In S. Falk, D. Rehfeld, A. Römmele, & M. Thunert (Eds.), *Handbuch Politikberatung.* VS Verlag für Sozialwissenschaften. https://doi.org/10.1007/978-3-531-90052-0_5

Mosquera, P. A., San Sebastian, M., Burström, B., Hurtig, A. K., & Gustafsson, P. E. (2021). Performing through privatization: An ecological natural experiment of the impact of the Swedish Free Choice reform on ambulatory care sensitive conditions. *Frontiers in Public Health, 9,* 504998. https://doi.org/10.3389/fpubh.2021.504998. eCollection 2021.PMID: 34136446 Free PMC article.

OECD. (2019). *Improving schools in Sweden report no 194.* OECD Education Working Papers strength through diversity's spotlight report for Sweden (online). https://doi.org/10.1787/19939019

Weingart, P., & Lentsch, J. M. (2008). *Wissen-Beraten-Entscheiden: Form und Funktion wissenschaftlicher Politikberatung in Deutschland.*

Production and Producers

A.1 What Is the Difference Between Basic and Applied Science, and What Is Their Respective Status in Society?

Basic science is a science field that *does not require immediate practical application of its findings*. Examples can be found in many different academic disciplines, ranging from physics, biochemistry, and other natural science disciplines to archaeology and art history, such as the exploration of Leonardo da Vincis painting techniques. Governments stimulate such activities in the conviction that such basic scientific activities are part of a good society and that they may or may not result in advances in an unpredictable way, sometime in the future. There is a tacit tolerance of the fact that a considerable proportion of basic research will never lead to practical applications, although a small proportion may lead to revolutionary new practical inventions, such as electricity, vaccines, antibiotics, and GPS (global positioning system). The fantastic success of the basic science tradition in the US has been built partly on this acceptance of the unpredictability of basic science.

There is a floating border between basic and applied science. In my imagination, while I was a child, basic research should be about chemistry, physics, mathematics, biology, and discoveries in nature. But the most important characteristic of *basic science* is probably that it is about *exploring the unknown*. This means doing basic research for its own sake, without a concern for immediate utility. This is a charming aspect of basic science, and the corresponding way of thinking has influenced my attitude to basic research positively, despite not doing much basic research. Basic science is at its best when it does not have to constantly prove utility. The most important groundbreaking discoveries have been made by scientists whose goal was to discover the unknown, not to be immediately useful to society. This means that a "playful attitude" might be an important component. One paradox is that mistakes could lead to important discoveries. One of the most well-known examples is Fleming's discovery of penicillin (see Tan & Tatsumura, 2015). Fleming

© The Author(s), under exclusive license to Springer Nature
Switzerland AG 2025
T. Theorell, *Underuse of Applied Science in Changing Societies*, SpringerBriefs
in Public Health, https://doi.org/10.1007/978-3-031-96391-9_2

one day left his laboratory for summer vacation and, by accident, left bacteria plates standing on a table without anybody attending to them. When he returned, the bacteria had been growing excessively, but in places where there was penicillin, there was no growth—a discovery of historical magnitude.

In a corresponding way, I define *applied science* as "science-driven efforts to describe and predict the outcomes of processes that are important in society." Applied science could have the role of a judge: When there are divided opinions about how to solve societal problems, results from impartial efforts in applied science should be one of the most important bases for decision making.

The borders between basic and applied science are fuzzy. I have spent nearly all of my scientific career in applied science in the fields of *psychosocial medicine* and *culture and health*. In some studies, I have worked closely with basic science, but the bulk of it has been in applied science.

My family history illustrates that the gap between basic and applied science exists. My father was a biochemist who was awarded the Nobel Prize in physiology and medicine in 1955. He knew all the technical aspects of how to do basic research, and he did not consider applied science, such as public health or epidemiological research, to be real science. "Whenever you need to use statistics to prove something, it is not science anymore" was a common statement in family dinner conversations. Despite this, research based on statistics has become my everyday life. The feeling of not being a "real scientist" has been with me all the time. My father, who was otherwise a considerate and reasonable person, was clear in his distancing from "science depending on statistics". Only late in his life, for instance, did he accept that there could be a causal relationship between tobacco smoking and lung cancer. The proof of this was mainly based on epidemiological statistics.

Thus, I have been aware of the distinction between basic and applied science since I was a child. And this is despite the awareness that the borderline between basic and applied science is fuzzy. "I am just pretending to be a researcher" is a sentence that I have carried with me throughout my career as a researcher, initially in clinical research while I was a clinically active physician, and then as a full-time researcher for several decades. My mantra tells me that I am not really a researcher— I am just moving around in the vicinity of science. That feeling is still a dominating one. I am not alone in this; the status difference between these two branches of science is reflected in many societal views.

In Nordic countries, population surveys and epidemiological research have been popular and attractive for researchers from the 1970s to the 1990s (Smith Jervelund & de Montgomery, 2020). This kind of applied research was regarded as important both by politicians and laymen. In addition, from 1964 to 1969, the Nordic countries established large cohort studies, which allowed studies of trends in these societies. Official cohort studies were repeated in the same way at regular intervals (in Sweden until 2006). High participation rates in high-quality population surveys confirmed strong trust among the public. This trust was also mirrored in research foundations providing high levels of financial support for this type of research.

The research community is also interested in the value of its work. Ratings have been published of how different kinds of research are valued among medical researchers, psychiatric patients, and lay people in general (May et al., 1986). Projects dealing with physical health, mental health, and resources for health care had the highest ranks, and there were surprisingly small differences based on age and gender. Politicians who were active during this period have recently affirmed that results from applied research were considered important in political decisions during that period (Karlsson, 2005).

Since the 1990s, governments have diminished their support for this kind of broad population research; this is paralleled by a dramatic lowering of participation rates in population surveys, from 80–90% down to 50% or even below. Part of the reason for this may have been that the methods introduced for scientific population surveys by sociologists and statisticians have been adopted by the sales industry. This means that survey technologies have been used to produce commercial sales campaigns. The population has been swamped by such sales-argument surveys. This may have reduced the willingness to participate in scientific surveys since such a massive number of surveys takes time and is perceived as benefiting only sales interests. And people in general may mix up serious scientific studies with commercial surveys intended to produce sales arguments. In this way, trust in scientific surveys has eroded. Another reason behind lowered participation rates may be the transition from physical person interviews to telephone interviews. In our country, this took place during the first years after 2000. Physical person interviews were judged to be too expensive. However, the motivation to participate and the reliability of answers are lower in telephone interviews than in interviews conducted in person. The response pattern may also change because of the transition (debate article by experts Amnå et al., Göteborgsposten, 2007).

In this phase, politicians still listened to researchers. A description of the clear influence of epidemiological research results on political health care decisions was published in 2005 (Karlsson, 2005). After this, however, the impact of scientific results seems to have decreased.

This development covering the whole population was relatively unique for Nordic countries, although large cohort studies have also been established in many other countries.

A.2 Conditions for Applied Research in Scandinavian Countries

When exploring the role of applied science in society, one must understand how those who produce the results in that discipline are recruited and what they think when they start a career. I will start using a myopic perspective, the stage for those who have been recruited to the general topic of psychosocial factors and health, and cultural activities and health in my own country, Sweden.

From the standpoint of scientific activity, Sweden was a favored country during the twentieth century. We managed to stay away from both world wars. Particularly during World War II, the development of science was halted from many points of view, particularly in Europe and Japan. Our country accordingly had advantages, and the Rockefeller Foundation and other scientific monetary beneficiaries sent considerable amounts of money supporting basic scientific activities in our country (Huldt et al., 2013), which accelerated the development of science here. At the same time, the political development in Sweden was favoring social democratic solutions in education, health care, sickness insurance, housing construction, and family policy. Accordingly, there was also an extensive need for applied science. Our social democratic governments decided to support their decisions by allowing Sweden to construct large representative population surveys informing society about economic development and working and housing conditions, to provide society with data facilitating wise decisions. Sweden is the largest Nordic country and was among the first in the world to establish such psychosocial databases.

The Level of Living Survey (LNU), initiated by the Swedish Institute for Social Research (SOFI) in 1968, and the Survey of Living Conditions (ULF), conducted by the Office for National Statistics (Statistics Sweden) since 1978, assess social and economic conditions to support research and policy development (https://rut. registerforskning.se/metadatakatalog/register/112f651e-96e2-4a0e-9e8d-2338f1f 9ba25). Since then, other high-quality Swedish population surveys have been launched, and there has been a similar development in other Nordic countries. An important reason for the success of such endeavors was that Nordic populations had trust in their government, so when interviewers were sent out for household interviews or people were asked to respond to questionnaires sent out by mail, the participation rate was very high, above 80%. The government also constructed powerful financial sources of public money for applied research. In the area of work environment research, a financial base for basic and applied research was constructed by means of a joint agreement between employer and employee unions. The conditions for societal applied research were therefore extraordinarily good during the 1950s to the 1990s in our country. This attracted many young Nordic and other foreign researchers, particularly from the US and other European countries, who wanted to spend time doing research in our country. It was also easy to attract research students from our universities. During this period from the late 1960s until the late 1990s, my research activities were primarily confined to medical research, casting light on the mechanisms underlying psychosocial stress (particularly at work) and various forms of illness, both psychiatric and somatic.

Another interesting feature in the first waves of Nordic representative population studies was that they were based upon personal contact between an interviewer, who had been trained in performing standardized data collection from randomly selected members of Swedish society. The state agency Statistics Sweden, which was responsible for this, employed and trained interviewers who lived in the same county as the interviewee. This means that the interviewer and interviewed shared knowledge and ideas about living area conditions. After three decades, the home visits were considered too expensive, and they were gradually replaced by telephone interviews. However, this also contributed to a rapidly falling participation rate, creating doubts about their representativeness. The Nordic epidemiological surveys of the population's living conditions were world famous and attracted researchers from around the world. This foreign input was a great stimulus for epidemiological research in Sweden (and other Nordic countries). An important question is, accordingly, whether one should go back to personal interviews as the primary method for collecting data about life habits and social conditions in the general population. This collection method is more expensive than telephone or computer. But if we get more reliable data, it may result in major gains in the future.

A.3 Factory Production of Doctoral Theses: The Driver's License for Scientific Acceptance

Notwithstanding, analyzing the pros and cons, it can be stated that during my years, there has been an enormous increase in the production of doctoral degrees. At the Karolinska Institutet, where I earned my doctoral degree in 1971, 100 doctoral degrees were awarded every year, but today the number is 380. There was thus an almost fourfold increase. The Karolinska Institutet is a PhD factory. Today, most of them are not physicians; they belong to other categories of research, such as biology, psychology, physical therapy, and epidemiology. This in itself is not a problem, but it is a problem that a lower proportion of physicians go through a research education. In addition, the students come from many different countries. We have many Chinese students, for instance, and from other countries in the East. That there are many foreign students is a good thing, but we also need to retain a high proportion of Swedes among our researchers.

However, other changes have taken place in the publication of original journal articles included in doctoral theses. Today, the most common doctoral thesis has four original articles published or to be published in international journals with independent reviewers. The external reviewers may be quite difficult to deal with. The student might even have to try a couple of different journals before getting them published. This can drag out for a couple of years, which is one of the threats to the four-year plan. But it also means that the product, the thesis itself, gets a quality check, which is more efficient than the one we had when I started.

As an example, at our university hospital in the Karolinska Institutet, I found a library with dissertations in medicine from the nineteenth century—among them a doctoral thesis from 1830. I read it with fascination because at the time, they had no external check, such as from a professor from another university who might approve or disapprove upon reading it. This doctoral thesis in orthopedics from 1830 was about one patient who came to the university hospital with a difficult problem in his left hip—a luxation that had happened some time before the consultation. And in the roughly 200-page thesis, the defendant writes about how they tried to pull that hip correctly, according to methods introduced by several famous orthopedists, in several attempts to fix the hip. But nothing worked. When they tried the final procedure, the whole leg broke instead. This man ended up not being able to walk at all.

I wrote a little play about this with some lyrics. When the patient lost his walking ability, I sang a song, based upon Lenski's aria from Tchaikovsky's opera *Eugene Onegin*, [translated] "Away, away went my ability to walk." This pivotal moment in *Eugene Onegin's* drama, where Lenski loses his beloved girl, mirrors his tragedy to a patient's loss of the ability to walk.

I was astonished by the poor quality of the thesis from the aforementioned nineteenth century occurrence and thought, "Today we have better quality." I assert this from experience during recent years as a retired professor on the final thesis review team with several other retired professors. I have seen a cascade of different kinds of doctoral theses in orthopedics, psychology, biochemistry, genetics, and social medicine. They have a higher quality today, yet something important has been lost in the construction of this kind of doctoral thesis, which usually has four parts, original articles published in international journals, combined with a summary, which the students are still supposed to write themselves.

The summary is less important than the journal publication, and the students often do not carry out the intellectual and analytical rigor required when constructing the whole thesis from the first to the last page on their own. I have observed that doctoral students are obliged to retain more of the do-it-yourself approach in several other parts of the world. In many universities in the U.S., this old-fashioned kind of doctoral thesis has remained prevalent. It is also found in many places in Great Britain, such as Oxford. But in most of Europe, they have the same system as Sweden—that is, according to the Bologna agreement, which was introduced in 1999 (Ministerial Conference Bologna, 1999). It is true that in the summarial approach used in most of Europe, the student has to produce his/her summary of the included (soon-to-be) published articles. This summary is intended to fulfill the autonomic role that used to be required in the more "total" production of doctoral theses of the past. It is still possible in Nordic medical faculties to produce a "total book" not solely comprising journal articles, but this is more common in qualitative studies, which are extremely rare in medical faculties in Nordic countries today.

But how did this apply specifically to how I selected my field of psychosomatic medicine? It does so in an interesting way. When I started my scientific career, psychosomatic medicine was a controversial field. The notion that psychological and social processes could give rise to bodily illness was facing skepticism. Therefore, choosing psychosomatic medicine for a research career required courage and tenacity.

In summary, there are many aspects of recruitment and conditions for young researchers to consider when choosing applied research, particularly in psychosocial medicine and culture and health. From an international perspective, there were favorable conditions in Sweden for this kind of research from the 1950s to the 1990s due to their nonparticipation in the world wars. The possibilities there for applied research (and basic research) were particularly good for physicians. Since then, the volume of research has expanded considerably, and researcher education has become much more formalized. In addition, our research recruitment has become much more international, and in general, the quality of research has improved, although the latter point may not be the opinion of all my colleagues. However, all my research colleagues would agree with me that we do more high-quality research today than researchers were presenting 200 years ago. Even though we produce increasing numbers of high-quality research and have more international contacts, the status of applied research is relatively low. It is impossible to classify all doctoral theses into either the basic or applied category because of the vague border between definitions. However, judging from the titles of doctoral theses at the Karolinska Institutet in the year 2024, a reasonable estimation is 50% for both categories. One way of summarizing the changes in recruitment to researcher careers during these years is to say that the quantity has increased, and that research education has become more like an extension of regular high school education. The chapter "Communication with Society" deals with the trust that the Swedish population has in various kinds of research.

Perhaps one other consequence of firmly establishing the new tradition of producing a solid article in a respected scientific journal as the main ingredient of a doctoral thesis, rather than a firm construction by the student of the total picture of the scientific problem, is that processes favoring this kind of integrative thinking have become less important. Might this decrease the trust among laymen? The answer, however, would be nothing but speculation on my part.

A.4 Changed Perspectives in Medical Applied Science Since the 1960s

When I started my career in the late 1960s, the population of researchers within society was much smaller than it is today, and there were many generally accepted principles regulating them. For instance, in the medical world, physicians used to be the ones conducting medical research. This is not the case today. Other occupational categories have been incorporated into medical research, to the extent that physicians are now the minority in the field.

In the 1960s and the 1970s, those who aspired to a position as chief physician somewhere in Sweden had to defend a doctoral thesis. This also used to be true outside of university hospitals. Chief physicians should have some knowledge of the field of research, but this is no longer a requirement for leadership, as it is frequently sufficient to be a licensed physician.

Another difference was that there was a lack of an elaborate system for judging scientific merit, except for an expectation for older researchers to make such assessments without formal criteria. Doctoral dissertations were evaluated using a four-tier subjective grading scale from *does not pass* to *laudatur* (highest distinction). When a dissertation was given a low grade, this impacted the whole career of that doctor, with a low grade for a dissertation being incompatible with a future career in research.

During my first few decades in the field, only assistants to full professors served as opponents and committee members for doctoral dissertation defenses. This is still true in the 2020s. In the beginning, they graded not only the dissertation but also the candidate's defense performance, using a grading system similar to elementary school and high school. It was like remaining a pupil in old schools. This more or less continues throughout the whole career in incremental advancements.

The everlasting evaluation process continued throughout the researcher's career. When they applied for a position as lecturer, assistant professor, or full professor, older professors were the ones who made the judgments. There were no numbers or formal criteria.

The scientific judges tried to be as objective as possible. In most cases, it did work, but sometimes it could also be quite wrong.

Today, when the society of researchers has grown so rapidly, there are many justifications for more objective judgment of their work, not least of which is that the number of assessments would be unmanageable without more or less mechanical criteria. The increase in volume is interesting from a historical perspective; the number of scientific journals recorded in the world between 1700 and 2001 grew from one to 11,000. After 2001, it exploded far beyond that. A problem that has been arising during recent years is that the publishers see articles in scientific journals as a source of money. They know that researchers want to (and are forced to) publish all the time. In a situation where you have an unlimited number of journals with unlimited space, it is always possible to find a journal that is willing to publish—if you are willing to pay. With enough funding, one could write endless articles and get them all published.

The judgment system, which involves the assessment of the scientific value of articles, is threatened by the combination of unlimited space and "paying for publication." If the journal earns money and wants to publish all the time, the whole objective judgment system is threatened. When external independent reviewers have assessed a manuscript submitted for possible publication as flawed and unsuitable for publication, the editorial office might decide to publish it anyway. In this way, bad research could be published today, simply due to the dominant influence of monetization—in other words, money rules. There is even an international list of so-called predatory journals and publishers called Beall's list, which researchers in the most prestigious universities are obliged to check before they decide to publish in a specific journal.

This means that there are many efforts to describe in more objective terms how well the publishing of research by a researcher or a group of researchers is working. This has resulted in the concept of the *impact factor*, defined as the average number of citations a journal achieves annually. This is applied to all the articles that an individual researcher publishes. The impact number is stamped on an article published by a researcher in a specific journal. Though this is crude and has been elaborated upon, the principle is sound.

One particularly difficult problem is the possible inclusion of many authors, and thus, the impact assigned to the individual researcher needs to be recorded differently depending on how many authors the article has and what the contribution of the individual authors may have been. A common solution is to give more weight to the first author. This has resulted in fights about who should occupy that favorable position.

Many scientific departments develop strategies for promoting their publications and use the system in an optimal and competitive way. This has another very strange effect, which is that the system changes at irregular intervals. If the department has used its strategy for many years, a change could mean that the newest criteria for getting good points may put all researchers in a more unfavorable position as changes are applied retrospectively. The opposite could also happen, resulting in a sudden improvement for all the employed publishing researchers in a scientific group. The only thing that counts in eternity and should count in the scientific world, therefore, is whether the research is good and makes a difference.

Serious journals could also use tricks to promote their journal. For instance, a journal editor could demand that the authors quote articles published in that journal. That is one way of collectively increasing the impact value of that journal. In a European journal that has used that strategy very consciously, the editor remained in that position for 20–25 years, and during that period, the impact value of that journal skyrocketed. The journal was very well edited, so this "manipulation" was only one of the reasons for the increase in impact.

Accordingly, the situation now in research is that we try to create objective criteria, relying very much on numbers. How many publications do you have in journals with high impact? This makes it difficult in the end to judge what is important. Accordingly, there are many threats to the validity and reliability of scientific publications. One of those that I have been discussing is very important, concerning how society uses science. If we go back to my situation, when I started in the 1960s and 1970s with a few journals and not many researchers, then it was easier perhaps to find more qualitatively reliable reports, which could be used by politicians.

Today, the situation is reversed: we have an abundance of publications and results, yet politicians are likely to pick those that align with their perspectives. This is probably true in all countries, and certainly in the United States. I had one experience that illustrates the relationship between society and researchers at the beginning of my career.

I was called by a scientific journalist from our biggest Swedish newspaper, and he said he had read an article in a scientific magazine—not a scientific journal, but a magazine—stating that people who are very sexually active are more likely to avoid having myocardial infarctions. That was a bold statement, and he wanted me to comment. I was, at the time, working at a cardiac intensive unit, and I said, "Oh wow." I should have said that this was, of course, rubbish, because you can never know which is the cause and which is the effect—are you sexually active because you are healthy, or does the sexual activity make you healthy? But instead, I said something that was not so cautious. I said, "There have been a lot of people who have suffered a myocardial infarction who believed that sexual activity would be forbidden for them for the rest of their lives. This, of course, is erroneous. If you take precautions, and if you do it in a friendly way, and so forth, you can stay sexually active."

The next morning, the biggest newspaper claimed that I, a 34-year-old physician, stated that "Sexual activity *soon* after a myocardial infarction is good for the patient." I was traveling by train to my job that morning, and I saw men reading newspapers and smiling at one another. I did not reveal who I was. Then I came to the intensive cardiac care unit that morning, and all the nurses, patients, and doctors looked at me with very curious faces.

That resulted in a call from our most famous, aggressive television journalist. He wanted me to join one of that evening's "sofa programs," where people sit and talk. I was, of course, enormously nervous. It was the most popular talk show at the time, and since Sweden had only two television channels at the time, it was something many people would have seen. I had a strong feeling that this journalist would try to get me to say things that I would regret for the rest of my life. However, I started thinking: "I know this subject much better than he does," realizing I could interrupt him if I needed to.

This was such a strong feeling. It was like somebody gave me the courage to manage this situation very well. But I do not believe this could have happened today in the same way, because we have a much more aggressive journalism climate. However, I came out of this without any problems. It was such an important experience for me. I think it does say something about the situation then vs. the situation today. Today, science can be used by anybody as an argument for heinous proposals, supported by some obscure scientific report somewhere. And the media (including social media) have a more aggressive agenda today than they had during the period when I communicated about sex after myocardial infarction. A respectful attitude from interviewers and researchers displayed through assertiveness in interview situations increases trust in applied science!

A.5 Financial Conditions

One of the most important differences for doctoral students today compared with the situation 30 or 40 years ago is that the financial conditions are much more clearly defined today than in previous years. Up to the 1990s, it was mainly up to the doctoral students themselves to arrange financial support during their research years. Particularly among my fellow doctoral students without a physician background, it was common to have no financial support at all for research. But this gradually changed, and finally, the universities were forced to arrange financial support for doctoral studies. One part of the background was that doctoral students were sometimes asked to do administrative work or to give lectures "as part of their research education," without payment. This could, of course, be labeled slavery. There were also problems on the opposite end—scientific institutions could be demanded to pay a salary to a doctoral student, a salary that had no coverage and could mean a severe strain on the institution. Finally, rules were formulated: The universities have to guarantee a salary for the doctoral student during a period that could be regarded as "normal" research time.

During the same period, research course requirements (e.g., statistical methodology, ethics, research design) were established, tailored to each doctoral student's needs. In other words, doctoral studies became formalized in several ways, and a normal research education period was defined as four years. This has mostly been translated into temporary research student positions. The universities are less and less willing to accept students outside the formal system. Since the number of students interested in starting a research education mostly exceeds the number of available positions, there is considerable competition. One problem with this development is that it has become increasingly difficult for clinically active physicians, nurses, psychologists, and physiotherapists to start a research career that builds upon observations in clinical work over a long period, and thus to be accepted as research students. The institutions do not dare to take on such people since they may be forced to employ them even if there is no money available.

In conclusion, I have outlined a gradual transition away from an informal, academically driven system, which used to allow men and women with extensive professional experience to explore ideas that had arisen from their collective experiences in applied research. The development has resulted in a more formalized system in which financial and administrative rules make it more difficult for those with occupational experience to translate that into applied research. Perhaps this is one reason laymen maintain a low level of trust in applied research.

References

Amnå, E., et al (2007, September 13). *En halv miljard av statens pengar riskerar att slösas bort (Half a billion Swedish crowns, 500 million dollars, run the risk of being wasted)*. Göteborgsposten.

Huldt, I., Normark, D., & Norrving, B. (2013). *Från läkarskola till medicinskt universitet: Karolinska institutets ledning 1953-2012*. Karolinska Institutet University Press. isbn:9789185565634.

Karlsson, M. O. (2005). Forskningsresultat omsatta till politiska beslut (Research results with implications for political decisions). *Socialmedicinsk Tidskrift, 2*, 142–148.

May, P. R. A., Smedby, B., & Wetterberg, L. (1986). Perceptions of the values and benefits of research. *Acta Psychiatrica Scandinavica, 74*.

Ministerial Conference, Bologna 1999. ehea.info

Smith Jervelund, S., & de Montgomery, C. J. (2020). Nordic registry data: Value, validity and future. *Scandinavian Journal of Public Health, 48*(1). https://doi.org/10.1177/14034948198985

Tan, S., & Tatsumura, Y. (2015). Alexander Fleming (1881-1955): Discoverer of Penicillin. *Singapore Medical Journal, 56*, 366–367. https://doi.org/10.11622/smedj.2015105

Research Students

B.1 What Attracts a Student to a Research Career?

The key research questions that interest me include: How do social and psychological processes get under our skin, and what can be done to prevent and cure these effects once they have presented themselves? Curiosity is my driving force. Before a student decides to enter a career exploring such questions, many other factors should be considered. Perhaps most people reading this would believe that if you have gone through a major dissertation test and achieved an academic doctorate, this automatically makes you a full-blown researcher ready to secure employment as a researcher. The path from dissertation to research professional does indeed proceed, but throughout a researcher's professional life, they learn to accept being repeatedly subjected to various examinations. The lifelong researcher must perpetually apply for money, constantly demonstrate intelligence, and regularly exhibit a high amount of activity—especially in research that is successful in obtaining grants from external funds. The one who fails at these essential self-marketing tasks runs the risk of being bypassed or excluded from the system. Once you have failed, the administration may ask you: "Why not seek a job as a teacher in high school?"

A doctoral degree remains a significant achievement, but recent developments reveal a diminishing regard for doctoral education. After completing a doctoral dissertation, choosing a research career is an esteemed path for a young scholar. It's common for a graduate to instead use that achievement as a mere CV highlight and opt for some other kind of career.

Accordingly, even those with a doctoral degree may have difficulties finding a good research-related job. The conditions for research students have varied. In the 1960s and 1970s, a physician could become a doctoral research student without having any financial support for it. For those who were physicians in university clinics, this was okay because doing research was part of the job, which meant doing it both during working hours and leisure hours. But clinical work with patients and

T. Theorell, *Underuse of Applied Science in Changing Societies*, SpringerBriefs in Public Health, https://doi.org/10.1007/978-3-031-96391-9_3

being on call were necessary activities performed while gathering data for their future doctoral dissertation. In the final stages of the dissertation work, there was a possibility to get research money, or even have a couple of months off to concentrate on finishing the dissertation, but that was not as easily arranged for nonphysicians doing medical research. In those cases, research was not included as a self-evident portion of one's professional life.

I would describe the attitude toward doctoral studies for physicians as very positive during my first years. This was also true among other medical faculties in our country. Although I have not assessed this in cross-country comparisons, it was my impression that this was also true in most other Western European countries and the United States. Producing a doctoral thesis was important—not only for oneself—it was required for those who wished to start a research career. It was also regarded as an important element of the development of the medical field that many physicians were knowledgeable in research methodology. And this was true not only at the bigger hospitals, but also in the countryside hospitals. Accordingly, there was a liberal attitude in the university clinics toward research, and there were no formal requirements to be accepted as a doctoral student except being a licensed physician. On the other hand, other professional groups in health care, such as registered nurses, physiotherapists, and occupational therapists, did not have access to a formal research career.

The research-friendly culture among physicians partly explains why there used to be few formalized research courses for doctoral students in medicine. It was considered sufficient to have been exposed to the research premises under the supervision of your peers. The student was expected to learn research work while doing research.

In humanistic and social sciences faculties, research education was more formalized. These had a very large number of regular students who wanted to become research students, but the universities could not accept all of them. Accordingly, they had to create limits and impediments, eventually organizing formalized requirements and formalized courses. Consequently, this formalistic aspect of research studies started to build up much more here than in the medical arena.

One of the differences between research students in medicine today and when I began my research studies was that before, even the financial conditions were unregulated. This meant that during intense phases of concentration on research, one may have even had to take several months off without payment. That was, of course, a hard reality. Today, the situation is different. Scientific institutions do not accept medical research students if there is no financial support for them. Rigorous applications for financial support must be formulated, and before a student is accepted, financial coverage must be guaranteed for at least four years. This, of course, is good for the students because they do not have to suffer financially, but on the other hand, it creates a very formalized, unspontaneous recruitment of medical students.

The contemporary formalization of a financial safety net for doctoral students has one other drawback. When a physician had been doing clinical work for many years, it used to be easy to mix research into it in informal ways. At present, it is more difficult to start a research career because it means a worsened financial situation— after all the rigorous procedures, the resulting research salary (if guaranteed) is low compared to the clinical one. This makes research education for a medical doctor unattractive. This has made those who have spent several years thinking about clinical work while treating patients less likely to contribute that insight to medical research.

Another new development has been restrictions surrounding financial support for research students that necessitate completion of a doctoral degree within four years. This creates problems when difficulties arise. Research is sometimes unpredictable. External events may also cause problems. For instance, the whole process may stop because of a pandemic, which makes it impossible to recruit patients. The financial support may melt down to nothing because it turns out that it is impossible to follow the research plan. This creates a rigid situation that is difficult to handle.

More specifically, one might ask to what extent doctoral students would engage themselves in applied research in psychosomatic mechanisms or research on arts and health. The topic is perceived as fascinating by some physicians, psychologists, and other health practitioners, but the status of such topics has been low in traditional academia. Basic science is considered high-status medical research, as has some applied science areas related to high-status care, such as cardiology, neurosurgery, hematology, and immunology. In psychiatry, pharmacological treatments have had a high status in Nordic countries, particularly in Sweden. The status of a specific subdiscipline mirrors the status of that discipline among laymen in general. Perhaps this is because easily defined "quick fixes" for health problems are favored over those that require long-lasting efforts by the individual, such as psychodynamic therapy or therapeutic exposure to the arts.

Summary During the decades I have focused on, the research career for physicians and other clinical workers has changed in many ways. There are several possible consequences:

(a) Due to financial arrangements, it has becomes significantly less likely for physicians with a solid clinical background to develop an appetite to pursue a research career in medical and caring research. Instead, students may decide at an early stage of their academic education whether they want to embark on a research career. In the long run, this is likely to benefit the areas of research that have a high status, such as neurosurgery and cardiology. As a speculation, I could add that this might decrease the trust that lay people have in applied research in medicine and caring—if those who have spent many hours in active patient care, developing advanced perspectives on improvements have difficultly getting into research, lay people might find that researchers are not exploring the fields of concern to the public.

(b) In the past, there has been a strong correlation between scientific status and the likelihood of being promoted in a clinical career. This link has been attenuated during recent years.

(c) Financial difficulties for research have created increasing dependence on external financial support, very often from industry with financial interests. This may have increased the risk of bias in choice of research areas and the research results themselves. Formulating grant applications has become an increasingly time-consuming activity that consumes energy that could be used for the research itself.

B.2 Recruitment of Research Students in Regular Medical Education

Students undergoing regular medical education to be licensed physicians are also exposed to scientific education. It is very common for medical students to be recruited as experimental subjects in scientific studies. Some of them end up as researchers themselves if the experiment turns out to be interesting for them. When I was planning an experiment at the beginning of my research career, I did what many researchers did—I turned to my own students. Students were indeed interested in research questions and therefore willing to participate; they also imagined that their relationship with the teachers would benefit from participating in experiments. However, when the experiments were potentially dangerous, this type of asymmetric power relationship could be ethically problematic.

When I started my research, the world of researchers was much smaller than it is today. Research was regarded as something exclusive, and society held us in high regard. Society had less insight into research than it does today. The strong feelings related to the Nazi medical experiments had resulted in the Second Nuremberg Court Trial, which ended in 1947 with the execution of seven physicians. The final consequence was that the World Medical Association in 1964 formulated the Helsinki Declaration, which made committees for research ethics mandatory for research in medical faculties in the whole world (Lövstrup, 2014). This process took many years, and when I started my research in 1969, there were no ethical committees at the Karolinska Institutet. These ethical oversight committees formed in the 1970s.

To specify why ethical committees are important for the credibility of applied research, I will describe in more detail the experiment I carried out on my students and myself. Neither I nor the students were at the time (the year was 1968) accustomed to considering ethical aspects of planned experiments. The experiment was designed to explore metabolic and subjective correlates of acute stress. The stress was mimicked with injections of rather high doses of adrenaline subcutaneously once an hour, starting at 08:00 during the day of the experiment, which was preceded by a control day without injections having plasma and urine samples drawn at regular intervals. That project would have been unlikely to be approved by a research ethics committee today. The effects of the high-dose adrenaline injections were pronounced. I remember that I felt that I should be angry, but most of the time, there was nothing to be angry about. However, when somebody in the environment did something innocent, I reacted disproportionately with anger. Luckily, nothing serious happened with the experimental participants despite strong cardiovascular effects.

Today, society has substantial insight into what is going on in research through ethical committees. Elected lay people from the political parties participate in committee meetings where all research applications are examined from an ethical point of view. This is the rule for all ethical committees in Nordic countries, with similar rules in European and Anglo-Saxon countries. There are also government representatives in research councils that determine principles in research politics (Lövstrup, 2014). Dangerous experiments were not so uncommon before the existence of ethical committees, and of course, we should be grateful that ethical examination is compulsory today.

Despite this major reform, there is an ongoing critique of the present organization. The critics argue that bold, uninhibited curiosity, which has sometimes been behind great discoveries, is inhibited in the present situation. A crucial point is that law experts have taken over the leading role in the committees, and this may also inhibit creative thinking in science. In addition, apart from lawyers and scientists, politicians are also elected to be members of scientific research committees. This raises the likelihood that political processes could influence decisions regarding what is ethically sound in science. Extreme political opinions may prohibit "unwanted" science via ethical committees! Therefore, the introduction of representatives from political parties (similar to politically appointed lay people in court trials) into ethical research committees has been criticized.

B.3 Who Are the Students Recruited for Medical Health Research? What Basic Training Did My Doctoral Students Have When They Came to Me? Transdisciplinary Subjects Have Been the Rule

In 1967, when I started my clinical education, research in medical faculties was mainly for medical doctors and students. It was not so common for psychologists, biologists, statisticians, and sociologists to do medical research, and this pertains both to basic and applied research. My own country was Sweden, but according to the contacts we had, the situation was very similar in the other Nordic countries as well as in Western Europe and North America. The percentage of physicians among research students in medical faculties has decreased. Among my students were 12 physicians, 10 psychologists, 11 licensed nurses, 6 behavioral scientists, 2 social anthropologists, 3 physiotherapists, 1 mathematician, 1 dentist, and 1 sociologist. My research areas have all been transdisciplinary, so this amount of diversity in the profession of doctoral students is not representative of the Karolinska Institutet or medical faculties in general. But the statistics indicate that physicians have become relatively uncommon among doctoral students.

Four of the doctoral theses that I supervised during the first years dealt with life events and their relationship with the onset of illness. This was also the topic of my doctoral thesis. Twenty-two of the theses involved psychosomatic medicine, which is a far-reaching subject—anything from endocrine stress reactions to the handling of patients and their relatives during treatment and rehabilitation. Sixteen dealt with different aspects of our work environment, how illness risks are arising in it, and how we can prevent illness development by improving the work environment. Two of them were directly focused on hospital care, while another dealt with cultural activities and how they affect us. The thesis subjects were difficult to separate from one another. Aspects of cultural activity have been studied both in psychosomatic and work environmental contexts, for instance. The distribution of student backgrounds mirrors the general situation among doctoral students in applied science at the Karolinska Institutet and other Nordic medical faculties during the decades I was active. Although medical applied science in general should show great gratitude to all those researchers who have a nonmedical background but have decided to contribute to medical applied science, there is a risk that the decreased participation of medical doctors in it might have a negative effect on people's willingness to accept results from applied medical science. But this is merely speculation from my part.

B.4 Supervisor and Doctoral Student

Although many years have passed since I completed my PhD studies, my memories of them are still clear. My supervisor was Richard H. Rahe, an American psychiatrist who devoted a lot of friendly time supervising me. After having collected data on life changes and their timing in relation to the onset of a myocardial infarction for patients who had been cared for in my hospital, I was responsible for the experiments with adrenaline injections described above. In examining patients who had suffered a myocardial infarction and had returned to their normal lives, I was also responsible for the collection of information in a longitudinal study, week after week, of life changes experienced during each follow-up week. The urinary output of adrenaline was monitored during these weeks. Rahe moved back to the United States from Sweden during my doctoral studies, and thereafter, I spent some time with him in California. The overall supervisory arrangement was ideal in the sense that he gave me a lot of time in the beginning, but in the final stages I had to be more independent.

As a supervisor myself, I spent a lot of time with my doctoral students. It still happened in one case that a doctoral student was dissatisfied with the amount of time I allotted to her, and she chose another main supervisor (although she kept me as a co-supervisor). Such conflicts are not frequent among doctoral students, and they reflect complicated situations. In most universities, there are no formal rules for how many doctoral students a professor is allowed to take. Some attractive professors could have a large number of students at the same time. Unfortunately, this means that some doctoral students feel neglected since their supervisor has very little time for them. In some universities, one tries to solve this problem by giving the student two or even three supervisors. This can create another problem: The supervisors might get into conflict with one another, forcing the student to choose between contradicting pieces of advice. During the long supervision process, it becomes evident to the student how the supervisor acts and vice versa. I have seen pronounced variations in doctoral student behaviors. Below, I describe three behaviors that could be of particular significance in delaying the work.

(a) **Anxiety and Protectionism**

Some doctoral students are afraid of communicating their results to their peers. This fear could be a realistic one since it occasionally happens that colleagues and even supervisors steal results. In the wider space of the research process, editors might delay publication of results because they have their own interests, such as publishing similar results before the author does. Although this is not a frequent phenomenon, situations have been described in which a research council rejects an application, and it turns out that one of the members of the assessment committee later publishes research triggered by that application. However, extreme fear of releasing results is always destructive since it is through communication between the doctoral student and the surrounding researchers that the doctoral student matures and understands the scientific dialogue. During discussions with other groups of researchers, ideas about how to interpret findings develop. Thus, communication with other researchers weighs more heavily than the risk of being robbed of ideas. Here's a wicked formulation: It may be those with only a few ideas of their own that are the most afraid of being robbed of ideas. Those with many ideas have nothing to fear. Such a liberal interpretation is, however, destructive if uninhibited. Researchers must guard some ideas before releasing them into the open. As a child, I heard biochemistry researchers discuss such concerns: "If patenting one's own results (for pecuniary reasons) becomes the dominant rule, international biochemical research collaboration will in the long run be destroyed."

(b) **Lacking Essential Researcher Qualities**.

Doctoral students may lack key research skills, including:

- Ability to creatively identify researchable problem areas and technical possibilities to attack those
- Assertiveness, stubbornness, and orderliness
- Ability to write pedagogically and linguistically well, as well as the ability to effectively present data orally
- Technical skills, for instance, in statistics, chemical analysis, and verbal analyses in qualitative interviews
- Language skills

It is the task of the supervisor to identify qualities in the doctoral student and to support the good qualities so that they develop. But sometimes the supervisor is not informed about the missing necessary qualities in the doctoral student.

One of my doctoral students had severe dyslexia, a fact that came to my attention after two years. During those years, texts were still produced on ordinary typewriters, and corrections were made with a pencil on paper. If the corrections are complicated with pieces that have to be moved, many misspellings and grammatical errors that are marked with different symbols, such as bubbles, arrows, and flags in different colors, the situation will finally be unmanageable for the dyslexic student. I noticed that I received manuscripts back with unchanged errors. If the supervisor knows about such a problem, an effective accommodation can be discussed and achieved. A person with dyslexia can have all the other qualities needed for a successful research career, but it does not work if the person tries to hide the problem.

(c) **Too High a Level of Ambition: "The Best Is the Enemy of the Good"**

This was frequently stated by my supervisor. This is also a difficult trade-off question. Of course, we shall strive for the best quality when we are doing research. But if a high goal induces an obsessive search for insignificant errors, the whole process may slow down. This may be the most central and complicated aspect of research supervision. Sometimes small details determine the conclusions of the results, but the totality is never lost.

On a higher societal level, the researcher community can be attracted to morbid processes because of an unreasonable level of ambition. Extreme competition may increase the risk of faked research results. At the beginning of my career, Nordic countries did not have so many examples of faked research results, whereas we read about this problem in the United States. One theory was that this was due to the high level of competition there. Today, false research results are reported to a much greater extent than previously reported. Indeed, there is more competition today. A cautionary note: I have not seen any scientific proof that a high level of competition increases the risk of faked results, but the assumption seems to be reasonable. The so-called Macchiarini disaster (see the chapter entitled "How Does Applied Science Operate?" on page XX) is an example of the effects of being in an atmosphere with extremely high competitive expectations. The university (here, the Karolinska Institutet) wants to see sensational discoveries, blurring judgment when faking adventurers enter the stage. A doctoral student may be drawn into such processes since he/she does not have the experience and tools to assess credibility.

Reference

Lövstrup, M. (2014). Helsingforsdeklarationen 50 år. Ur nazismens grymheter föddes forskningsetiken. (Helsinki declaration. Research ethics born from the cruelties committed by the Nazi government). *Läkartidningen, 111.*

How Does Applied Science Operate?

C.1 How Is Applied Science Operating? One Example from a Mix Between Basic and Applied Science—The Job Strain Story

Why do young students enter and stay in a medical research career in our country? The reasons for entering and staying in applied medical research may have changed between the 1970s and the 2020s. In psychosocial medicine and culture-health research, a primary motivation was to explore how social and psychological processes can "get under the skin" of people, leading to illness. These findings should have a major impact on political decisions with long-term implications. Understanding the mechanisms that link psychosocial to somatic processes is significant because physical illnesses are more readily accepted as grounds for health insurance, sick role recognition, and allocation of health care resources in countries and regions. Accordingly, since it has been proven that psychosocial processes contribute to the development of myocardial infarction, stroke, high blood pressure, dementia, and some forms of cancer, it has impacted public attitudes regarding these processes—we take them more seriously than we did 50 years ago.

I have been involved in an international scientific effort to explore the relative importance of the psychosocial work environment as it relates to illness development. One of the goals was to formulate a theoretical model that could be acceptable to most researchers and could also be useful to society in most countries. It should be useful in the sense that it could apply to real-world work settings, which contribute to both mental and physical illness. If it turned out to have explanatory and robust value, there should be biologically plausible mechanisms that could explain the associations. Although there is certainly no total agreement about the resulting model's usefulness, it has become widely used both in research and in practice in many countries. It has also stimulated the development of similar but competing theoretical models. The model's theoretical relationship to individual and

T. Theorell, *Underuse of Applied Science in Changing Societies*, SpringerBriefs in Public Health, https://doi.org/10.1007/978-3-031-96391-9_4

environmental factors is presented in Fig. 1. It builds upon the idea originally formulated by Karasek (1979) that excessive psychological demands (*high demand*) could give rise to illness if, at the same time, the individuals in the workplace cannot exert control over their job situation (*low control*). This is labeled the *job strain* model.

Figure 1 illustrates the complicated interaction between the *job strain* environment (in this case, high demands in relation to low control), the *individual program*, which is built by genetic factors and previous experiences, and *reactions* to the environment. Three kinds of reactions can be identified: behavioral, psychological, and physiological. We are aware of some of these reactions, and we can also train ourselves as well as the workplace to become aware of them. A psychologist can help us become aware of our psychological reactions. A physiotherapist may teach us awareness of how we move our bodies in stressful situations, and by means of physiological equipment, we can also train ourselves to become aware of how our blood pressure, blood glucose, sweating, heart rate, and additional physiological functions react in different kinds of situations. The study model identifies the psychological demands coming from the work organization and suggests strategies that employees may engage in to exert control over those demands. The degree to which employees can obtain support from the organization (social support) is also a significant positive factor that can decrease illness risk.

The *job strain* model illustrates how one kind of question can stimulate a large group of researchers worldwide to focus their efforts on developing a researchable question: *How* can psychosocial conditions in one sector, working life, influence the pathogenesis of an important life-threatening disorder, myocardial infarction, or ischemic heart disease? Furthermore, if a relationship is proven, what importance does that potential relationship have on a societal level? How important is it in comparison to other kinds of risk factors? And finally, to what extent are these other risk factors related to the psychosocial conditions at work?

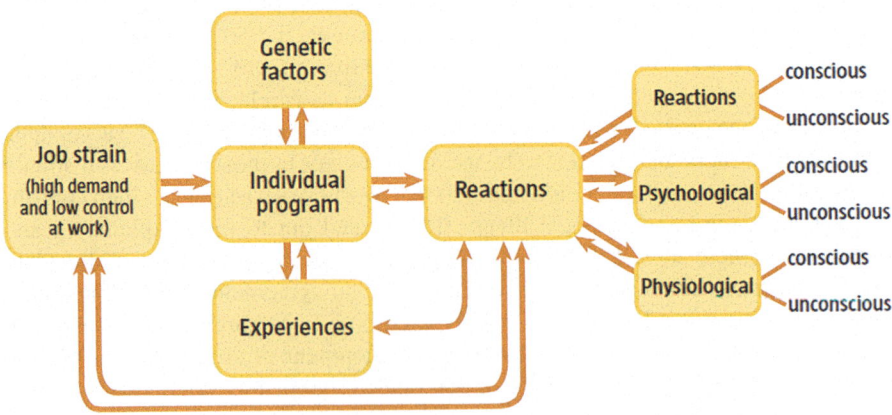

Fig. 1 Job strain relationships (Credit: Annika Röhl, 2025)

To conclude that psychosocial processes contribute to the development of myocardial infarctions, researchers have been forced to develop several scientific tools created in basic science, such as:

• **Mathematical models**: In epidemiological science, methods have been developed that make it possible to calculate the likelihood that a previously healthy individual with assessed scores on several risk factors, such as smoking, age, sex, blood lipid profile, blood pressure, and psychosocial risk, will develop a myocardial infarction. Thus, the effort is made to adjust for other "accepted" risk factors when the "independent" risk associated with the psychosocial factor itself is identified. This statistical technique, which has been established from basic science, is multiple logistic regression. In addition, one must find techniques for gathering and harvesting data from thousands of individuals and follow them over time, simply because, fortunately, myocardial infarctions are not so common among previously healthy people. Accordingly, researchers have established large collaborative networks to be able to recruit hundreds of thousands of participants. The examination of these kinds of questions demands the participation of expertise from cardiology, physiology, and epidemiology.
• **Psychosocial theoretical models**: Developing models that accurately reflect real-world conditions requires the participation of sociologists, psychologists, and occupational health scholars to ensure credibility and relevance.

It started with a sociologist. In psychosocial job research, the term *job strain* was introduced by the American sociologist Robert Karasek (see Karasek, 1979; Karasek & Theorell, 1990). The proposition is that high psychological *demand*, which people in general associate with stress, would have worse psychophysiological consequences when it is unlikely that a worker is able to influence *control* over their work. This *demand-control* theory was tested by means of a small number of work environment questions that working people were asked. Between 1978 and today, research on the demand control theory has been extensive. At first, the relationship was studied between working in a job with high psychological demands and low control, job strain, on one hand, and the risk of developing an objectively defined illness outcome, myocardial infarction, on the other hand. When subjects describe psychological symptoms related to the work environment, bias may play a role. Initially, patients who had suffered a myocardial infarction were asked about their working conditions, and their responses were compared to those of subjects without myocardial infarction in case-control studies. Such studies were criticized because feeling ill because of heart disease might create a biased view of the working conditions. Therefore, in the next step, prospective studies were performed, in which large groups of working people were asked initially about working conditions. They were then followed for several years. After adjusting for several other risk-related factors—age, sex, blood pressure, smoking habits, educational level, and initial blood lipids—it was possible through multiple logistic regression to calculate an independent risk associated with job strain.

After a long period of skepticism among colleagues, it was finally accepted that working in job-strain conditions is associated with approximately 30% excess risk of developing a myocardial infarction (acute ischemic heart disease episodes). This corresponds to an *attributable fraction* for job strain in relation to ischemic heart disease of 6%. This means that after adjustment for other relevant factors, 6% of such disease episodes among working people could theoretically be prevented if all job strain could be eliminated. Six percent may not sound like a strong effect, but on a population level, it would mean that in Sweden, 600 male cases of myocardial infarction would be prevented each year. This information can be combined with findings from research on other outcomes, such as psychiatric depression, stroke, diabetes, and musculoskeletal disorders. If the effects of job strain on all these outcomes are added to one another, it becomes evident that the societal impact of job strain on occupational health is substantial (Theorell, 2020, 2023). There are also other working conditions related to work organization that add to the total burden, such as shift work, extremely long working hours, and noise.

During these years, competing psychosocial models were also developed, such as the Effort Reward Model (Siegrist, 1996), which postulates that perceived high effort should be matched with positive reward. If there is a poor match, or an *effort-reward imbalance*, an increased risk of developing a myocardial infarction arises. The job strain and effort-reward models overlap to some extent, but they supplement one another, so combining them improves the prediction of illness risk. Another model for assessing psychosocial working conditions is the so-called demand-resources model, which is more flexible than the other two models and considers more individual characteristics (Demerouti et al., 2001).

While large-scale epidemiological studies on myocardial infarction risk were performed, studies of relevant physiological mechanisms, mainly in the field of stress endocrinology, were also done. In one of the first studies, we followed male employees in several occupations every quarter through a working year, collecting blood samples, blood pressure measurements, and questionnaire data about psychological demands and control at work as well as sleep quality. We were able to show that blood pressure levels during working hours were higher, sleep quality was worse, and anabolic hormone (testosterone) levels were lower in these men when the job strain was at its highest levels. This study gave a hint that periods of job strain cause energy mobilization (blood pressure elevation) and, at the same time, suppress regenerative functions. That combination is functional in an acute situation, but if it lasts for long periods (weeks), it may cause bodily harm. A large number of studies of the relationship of biological factors to the job strain model have been published, and although there have been conflicting findings there is evidence to say that long-lasting job strain influences stress hormones, immune reactions and cardiovascular functions via stress mechanisms and that it is also true that the body's defense is weakened during such periods. This increases the risk of developing many kinds of illnesses, for instance, depression, cardiovascular conditions such as myocardial infarction, and musculoskeletal diseases such as neck pain. A more detailed physiological explanation follows (from Theorell, 2009):

> One of the central parts of the stress reaction is the Hypothalamic Pituitary Adrenocortical (HPA) axis extending from the hypothalamus to the adrenal cortex… If the organism interprets the situation as energy demanding, a chain of reactions starts, resulting in raised blood

concentration of corticosteroids. In many ways, these corticosteroids help the organism sustain its fight in a stressful situation. In the acute situation, this is purposeful since the release of energy is facilitated by mobilization of fuel for energy-requiring actions (carbohydrates and free fatty acids), and there is retention of salt and fluid, which may otherwise get lost in an uncontrollable way in a physically demanding situation. There is also a temporary inhibition of acute inflammatory reactions. However, if the stressor is long-lasting (for instance lasting for weeks or months) those same effects may be damaging...

The "good" counterbalancing system, an anti-stress system which protects from adverse effects of long-lasting stress, is labeled the HPG (Hypothalamic Pituitary Gonadal) axis with the same levels as the HPA axis, but in the HPG, the involved actors range from the hypothalamus through the pituitary to the gonadal glands...The male testes and the female ovaries are the end organs of the HPG axis. They represent the extreme of the formation of new cells, namely, reproduction. "Building a new human individual" is, of course, the most pronounced *anabolic/regenerative activity* that the body can be involved in. Building new cells and repairing worn-out tissues is closely related to this, however...The two forces, *energy mobilization* and *regeneration*, are balancing one another on all levels of the HPA and HPG axes.

In all bodily organs, cells are being worn out and have to be repaired or replaced. In some cell systems, this is a rapid process (days or weeks, such as in mucosa, skin, and white blood cells), whereas in other systems it is slow (months, such as in the skeleton)... Testosterone and oestrogen, as well as their precursor DHEA-s (dehydroepiandrosterone sulphate), are examples of corticosteroids with mainly anabolic/regenerative function... There is a balance between the HPA axis and the HPG axis. This means that the HPG axis tends to lower its activity when the HPA axis has maximal activity (in stressful situations). But it also means that damaging effects of long-lasting stress can be dampened by a high activity in the HPG axis.

A *translation* of the physiological dimensions to the practical dimensions in the workplace would be:

Excessive psychological demands—HPA axis

Control at work—HPG axis

Support at work—HPG axis

Many other scientific questions had to be illuminated during the process. Can we eliminate subjective components in the assessment of job strain by avoiding the use of self-administered questionnaires? This was important since the focus was on work organization. Yes, one way of doing it is to construct Job Exposure Matrices (JEMs) for the assessment of psychological demands and job control. The average ratings of these parameters for defined groups (for instance, all plumbers above a certain age) are calculated from a population study. In another group without individual ratings, the average can be used as a proxy for everybody's situation in that particular group. Another methodology that was tested was to train observers to rate these dimensions in different workplaces. It is meaningful to try to assess as honestly as possible the way in which the work is organized. If the organizational factor is related to illness risk, this may provide a recipe for the improvement of worker health. The subjective component is also significant, but individual response patterns require another set of interventions than do work organization problems, although there is, of course, an overlap. Summaries of findings from comparisons between more objective and more subjective measures of the work organization have shown that the different sets of measurements are related to the outcome, myocardial infarction, with similar excess risks. This pertains particularly to the control dimension, which is less influenced by subjective perspectives than the demand dimension.

We also explored the possible significance of genetic makeup. We used the Swedish twin registry for this. Genetic make-up could explain part of the self-reported work environment and also the self-reported depression score. There could be a possibility that such associations, both on the explanatory and the resulting side, could explain away the job strain relationships. The results from our twin study (Theorell et al., 2016) indicated that self-rating of depressive feelings did have a moderately strong association with genetic makeup, and genes also influenced the way in which individuals described their demands and control at work. However, a cross-analysis indicated that these associations could not explain away the association between demand and control on the one hand and depression on the other hand. Part of the division between genes and environment is indeed partly a fallacy since genes (for instance, genes related to stress reactions) can be activated and deactivated by the environment. A stressful environment can make stress-related genes sensitized, and a stable, supportive environment can make them less sensitive. Parts of the gene chemistry regulating this have been clarified. This represents the growing scientific field of *epigenetics*.

The job strain model has also been used in practical work with work organizations. Excessive psychological demands are common in modern working groups. In summary, the complicated process that was established for assessing job strain's potential significance for the development of ischemic heart disease involved hundreds of scientists and hundreds of thousands of study participants. Results from studies were discussed at congresses and published and debated in journals. Negative and positive findings were published, confirming or rejecting the relationship. The magnitude of the association was also discussed extensively, as well as pathways from the job strain situation to the illness. The discussion was particularly hot regarding the mechanisms—did job strain stimulate people to adopt an unhealthy lifestyle (such as smoking and lack of physical activity), or was the effect due to direct physiological stress mechanisms? If the direct mechanism is more important, the interventions should be focused on stress mechanisms related to job strain. If lifestyle is an important intermediary type of factor, the emphasis should instead be on how job strain stimulates adverse behavior. The truth seems to be, not unexpectedly, that both pathways are important.

The job strain story illustrates how the scientific community works when it wants to find a useful concept that could guide societies in how to organize work. That is far from a common belief among lay people—that scientific statements are only biased statements from one group in society. What lay people do not always know is that the whole job strain process that I described is specifically about *avoiding bias*. There is a never-ending process in which scientists discuss the *real* description of reality. In this long chain, all the conditions that may be of importance are weighed against one another. It also illustrates that different kinds of specialists have to collaborate, as well as that an even larger group of working people has to participate in a systematic gathering of data.

Another common misconception is that scientists only produce books that are stored on a bookshelf and have nothing to do with the real world. Nothing could be more wrong. The scientific findings from studies of how psychosocial working conditions relate to illness risks are based upon real people's descriptions of their real world and how that relates to illness outcomes. The job strain concept has been used in the construction of national surveys of working conditions in several countries, such as the Nordic countries, France, Great Britain, the Netherlands, the USA, and Belgium.

Of course, there are situations in which the scientific process goes astray, and the reason for that could either be mistakes that scientists make or crimes against scientific rules. But the vast majority of scientists are honest people who try their best to find the truth. This is the basic idea behind science, including applied science. Let us look at the recruitment for applied science.

If a larger proportion of the general population were more knowledgeable about the scientific goals and ways of operating, it would probably benefit trust in applied science.

C.2 Research on the Connections Between Music and Health

Another example (in which basic science was intertwined with applied science) in more recent years is when I collaborated with Fredrik Ullén, a professor of neurobiology at the Karolinska Institutet as well as a professional classical pianist. His research group was able to conduct a series of studies based on the Swedish Twin Registry. This research was supported by the Tercentenary Fund, which provides larger multi-year grants.

Firstly, the Twin Registry can be used as any population survey. In these types of studies with complete twin pairs, one twin is randomly excluded to avoid erroneous associations in the analyses. By doing this, the studies function like regular population surveys. Secondly, one can, of course, utilize the opportunity to determine the extent to which observed associations are genetically determined.

It is widely agreed that musical experiences can evoke various emotions and amplify existing emotions when one listens to music. However, a somewhat different question arises: Could repeated musical experiences influence our emotional "skill," that is, our ability to differentiate, label, and convey emotions in the long term?

Being able to distinguish, interpret, describe, and convey emotions is crucial for effective communication with others. Someone who, for example, cannot differentiate between their own anger and sadness may struggle to correctly interpret such emotions in others. Sad feelings might be misinterpreted as anger. This miscommunication can lead to emotional problems and unnecessary conflicts. This lack of emotional processing ability is known as alexithymia. Usually, alexithymia is measured using questionnaires, which work well for non-psychiatric populations.

Alexithymia was the subject of several sub-studies in a Swedish music project funded by the Tercentenary Fund called "The Musician Human."

In the first group of studies, the aim was to investigate the strength of the association between cultural activities, especially musical ones, and alexithymia. As a measure of musical activity, participants provided self-estimates of the number of hours they had spent playing musical instruments or singing during different age periods (6–11, 12–17, and 18 or older). The participants were between 27 and 54 years old at the time of the survey. The responses were collected through a web-based questionnaire. The survey also included questions about other cultural activities, such as writing, visual arts, theater, and dance, with participants rating their involvement on a seven-point scale, from 1 (no activity at all) to 7 (professional performances with media reviews).

Alexithymia was more common among men than women (Theorell et al., 2014). However, the analyses of the associations between the number of music hours and alexithymia revealed that the associations were of similar magnitude for both genders. If the musical activity occurred in an ensemble form, this also contributed to the associations. Comparing the upper and lower thirds of the distributions for the number of music hours, and considering ensemble participation, those who played the least and had no ensemble experience had nearly half a standard deviation higher alexithymia scores (meaning more difficulties in handling emotions) compared to those who played the most and had ensemble experience. The associations with the level of success in music activities (according to a seven-point scale) were of similar magnitude and direction as those with the number of music hours.

The genetic analyses showed that the entire association between the number of hours of musical practice and the degree of alexithymia could be explained by genetic factors contributing to both alexithymia and the number of music practice hours. When combining the associations in a common model, the number of music practice hours no longer had an *independent* association with emotional processing ability. Approximately 30% of the variation in alexithymia was attributable to genetic influences, which can be considered a relatively low value compared to what is typically found in twin studies for physical and psychological variables.

In conclusion, we cannot say that actively playing music causes good emotional coping ability. We can only say that these factors are associated with each other (as described above, this was a disappointment to me!) It may sound pessimistic from a public health perspective, but to assess such aspects, we need to conduct robust intervention studies with proper evaluations. The fact that the associations are influenced by genetics means that large groups must be used to establish causality. It is essential not to have unrealistic expectations about what we can expect. One should also bear in mind that genetic factors can confound population surveys. Parents largely choose activities for their children, which results in correlations between genetic and environmental factors in population surveys, complicating the analyses. Still, it can be argued that a well-developed society should support individuals with exceptional emotional abilities. If there are resources available to help these individuals develop their musicality, it could be beneficial not only for themselves but also for society. This does not contradict the idea that people with less natural inclination for music can also benefit from musical experiences, and society has a responsibility for this as well. Tone-deafness is very rare; according to several measurements, it occurs in about 4% of the general population.

In two other studies, we explored the connections between alexithymia and other cultural activities in the same dataset. In the first study, we asked whether each of the cultural activities, such as writing, music, visual arts, theater, and dance (using the seven-point scale), could statistically explain any part of the variation in alexithymia independently. Additionally, we investigated whether simultaneous participation in multiple cultural activities would lead to even better emotional coping abilities (Lennartsson et al., 2017). Does being a writer, musician, and visual artist in the same person make them extraordinarily "better at emotions"?

The results from 2279 men and 3152 women showed that both writing and music abilities had independent statistical predictive value for alexithymia scores, regardless of the other activities (and also independently of age and education) for both men and women. The more professional a writer/poet or musician, the lower the alexithymia score (indicating better emotional coping). For men, visual arts, and for women, theater, also had similar independent predictive value for alexithymia. The answer to the second question was that individuals who scored high in a couple or several cultural activities (*multicultural*) were especially good at handling emotions.

Roughly, the difference between amateurs and the completely culturally inactive in each of the four cultural activities—writing, music, visual arts, and theater—corresponded to about one-quarter of a standard deviation on the alexithymia scale, both for men and women. Regarding the cumulative cultural activities, the difference between the top and bottom "culture" thirds was almost half a standard deviation on the alexithymia scale. Thus, there was evidence to suggest that involvement in multiple cultural areas was associated with particularly good emotional coping abilities.

When we talk about differences of about one-quarter to one-half of a standard deviation, some may argue that these are small differences. That is true. For example, the level of musician experience explains only a small percentage of the variation in the degree of alexithymia in the population. However, when discussing these associations at the population level, it corresponds to many individuals in the population.

Why is the discussion about music's potential effect on emotional ability important from a societal point of view?

In many countries in the world, there is a discussion regarding the effectiveness of the school system. In particular, skills in mathematics are considered central in contemporary and future societies. In Sweden, mathematical skills in high school students have deteriorated during recent years, according to PISA assessments. There could be many underlying reasons for this deterioration, but one that is frequently mentioned is unrest in the classroom. Regardless of what researchers mention, politicians favor one solution, which is to expand the number of lessons per week in mathematics. This time space must be created at the expense of other subjects, and the solution is frequently more hours of mathematics and fewer hours of arts education, for instance, music. A large practical experiment in Switzerland (Weber et al., 1993) lasting for three years with 52 classes distributed throughout Switzerland, however, showed that an increase in the number of hours of music per week benefits the social atmosphere in the classroom and that this benefits the learning atmosphere. The 52 classes were randomly assigned to an experimental and a control population. Music teaching was expanded in the experimental group with a slight decrease in the number of lessons per week in mathematics and language. Assessments of knowledge and social atmosphere were made regularly in both populations. The observed benefit in social atmosphere scores in the experimental population may explain why a reduction in the number of mathematics hours per week did not lead to deteriorated skills in mathematics. The same observation was made for language: A reduced number of language hours per week because of the increased music teaching, which did not result in worse knowledge of language. Similar studies with similar findings have been performed in Australia and the UK. Increased training in socioemotional skills by means of music training may improve the quality of the learning environment, not only during the music lessons.

We have made a related observation in my own research (Lindblad et al., 2007): Pupils in the fifth and sixth grades in a regular school in Stockholm were assigned to one of three groups:

Intervention A: One extra hour of music per week during the whole school year. The teaching of music was designed with a specific goal: to stimulate cohesiveness. This means that elite performance was not a primary goal. All the pupils could contribute, for instance, by singing or using simple drums. Rhythm was an important aspect.

Intervention B: One extra hour of computer training during a whole school year was introduced for this group.

Control group: Nothing extra was added. The pupils had the regular curriculum, which also included some music.

In all three groups, saliva cortisol was assessed at lunch time on three occasions, at start (August) and end of the autumn semester (December), and finally at the end of the spring semester (June). The results (Fig. 2) showed that there were no changes in saliva afternoon cortisol concentration in the control group, from start through middle to the end of the school year. In the computer group, there was a statistically insignificant increase in saliva cortisol concentration in December, but in June, the cortisol levels were the same as in August. In the music group, there was a significant decrease in afternoon cortisol levels, which is probably explained by a calming of the atmosphere in the classroom. Of interest was that this decrease did not happen rapidly—the extra music teaching had to last for a whole year before the change was observable. The experiment was relatively small and is in need of replication by other researchers. But it may confirm that this type of cultural input could contribute to an improved learning atmosphere. And it may also be one reason for the observation in the larger Swiss experiment that expansion of the room for *social music*

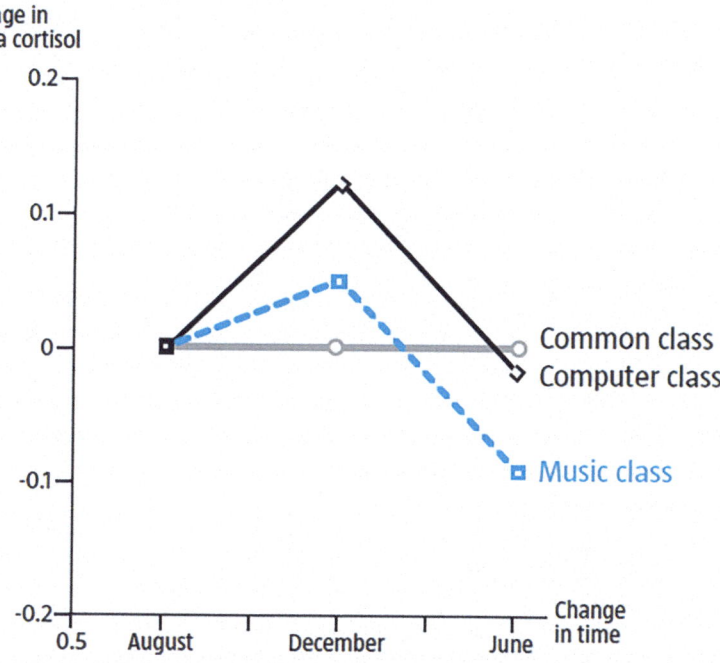

Fig. 2 Changes in saliva cortisol concentration in children participating in the year-long music experiment in a regular school in Stockholm (Credit: Annika Röhl, 2025). Blue: extra music one hour/week during the whole year (music class). Black: Extra computer teaching one hour/week during the whole year (computer class). Grey: Regular school year. Change in mean saliva cortisol (nmol/l) from start of fall semester (August = 0) to end of fall semester (December) and end of spring semester (June) in three experimental groups. Dots show mean changes (nmol/l)

training could be instituted at a small expense of the number of math and language lessons without adverse effects on results.

Socioemotional skills are important. If people have physical and cognitive skills but lack socioemotional ones, it is very difficult to build functioning societies. In an increasingly complex world, collaboration in groups is extremely important. The skillful use of cultural subjects at school not only creates a good learning environment, but it also contributes to structuring the brain in growing children in such a way that they will function socioemotionally better in a future society.

The training of musical skills in childhood can result in anatomical changes in the growing brain, supposedly related to socioemotional skill, as illustrated by another study performed by Ullén's group (De Manzano & Ullén, 2018). They examined the brains of nine 27- to 54-year-old monozygotic twin pairs that differed (pair discordant) concerning piano playing in life; one of them had spent more than 1000 hours practicing piano playing while their twin had spent zero hours. The research question was: Do the brains in the playing and nonplaying twins differ? This is important because monozygotic twins have identical genes. Accordingly, a difference in brain development across the life span in these twin siblings could not be solely genetically shaped. Magnetic resonance imaging showed that there were several types of differences between the brains of the playing and non-playing twins: Firstly, there were differences that had to do with the motoric functions related to the playing itself. For the pianist, the right hand's fingers (left side of the brain) are particularly important, and that part of the brain was also more developed in the playing twin. Secondly, structures related to hearing and transforming musical input in the auditory (hearing) cortex, as well as in a network of brain functions related to emotional translation of the music, were more developed in the playing twin. Thirdly, the structure linking the left and right brain hemispheres (corpus callosum) was more developed in the playing twin. This is important not only because coordination between left and right is very important in instrument playing, but also because this structure is important for socioemotional skill in general. Accordingly, the findings in this study give concrete support to the idea that music training can stimulate the development of socioemotional skills. And we can even see objectively the anatomical changes associated with this! Such knowledge has never existed before. Societies should be more interested in this than they are. This is one of the reasons why I worry about society's unwillingness to pay attention to applied science, such as the Swiss experience of increased music teaching at school and our own music experiment in Stockholm. Both of these experiments showed that carefully chosen classroom music teaching (which favors togetherness) can benefit the learning environment, which could in its turn benefit emotional and social competence in children, not only at school but also when these children become adults. What about a possible future decrease in crime rates and an increase in collaborative skills?

C.3 Publishing Results that Go Against One's Own Bias

In research, there are strict rules that all researchers must adhere to for science to maintain its position among societal institutions. Whenever any form of research misconduct is revealed, the entire research community loses credibility, and the role of science as one of the functions entitled to societal financial support is threatened.

A fundamental duty of a researcher, therefore, is to publish results that contradict his/her own hypotheses, rather than only confirming his/her own theories. One probably does not become a mature researcher until one has gone through this kind of trial. On at least two occasions, I have published research that showed I had been wrong in my theories. So, in that regard, I am a mature researcher!

The first time I had to go against my own hypothesis in a publication was after I had published my doctoral thesis, which, among other things, showed that patients who had recently experienced a heart attack reported an unusually high number of life events in the months before their heart attack. After completing my thesis, I had the opportunity to follow approximately 8000 construction workers over time. They were asked to fill out a questionnaire about life events they had experienced in the past year. We then followed them for a couple of years. The hypothesis was that construction workers who had a heart attack during the follow-up year would have experienced a large number of significant life events the year before the study. However, this turned out not to be the case. Instead, a specific type of life event—increased job responsibility—was more common among construction workers who had a heart attack during the follow-up year compared to other construction workers. Moreover, when we followed the participants over two years, we could also demonstrate that work-related stress, even if not considered as specific events, was more common among workers who had a heart attack during follow-up compared to others. Therefore, a large number of significant events, in general, were not the decisive factor, but rather the type of events the participants had experienced. These studies on life changes and heart disease from our group have been summarized (Theorell, 2022).

There were thus two main hypotheses. The first hypothesis emphasized the importance of significant energy mobilization when many events occur around the same time. If this mobilization is prolonged, the risk of developing illness in general increases. This can be seen as a general stress theory. Richard Rahe, my supervisor during my thesis work, was a strong proponent of this theory. The second hypothesis emphasized the significance of what life events mean for an individual's situation—only events that pose a threat can accelerate the onset of diseases. The results of the prospective study of construction workers must be considered as supporting the second hypothesis, not the one that was my own and Rahe's.

However, Rahe had also stated that the group of individuals accustomed to life changes from time to time, and who therefore expect a constant demand for adaptation to new circumstances, differs from the group of individuals leading a life with few events. In the former group, significant changes may be required to affect health, while in the latter group, fewer life events are needed for health effects. According to this reasoning, it is the dynamics that matter, rather than the absolute level during a specific period—it is necessary to observe the pattern over time. There is also a pronounced difference between individuals concerning the propensity to react with an increase in adrenaline excretion when subjects experience life changes. In an early study of patients who were back to their ordinary life after having experienced a myocardial infarction, we followed the number of life changes every week. There was a clear group relationship between the amount of life change during a given week and the amount of urinary adrenaline excretion during the last day of that week; the higher the life event score, the higher the adrenaline excretion. But this explained only 10% of the total variance on the group level. When everyone was analyzed separately, it was found that one-third of the subjects were high, one-third moderate, and one-third had no correlations at all between life change amount and adrenaline excretion during a given week (Theorell et al., 1972). It appears some individuals are highly sensitive to the kinds of life changes that we studied, while others are much less responsive.

Does this have any significance? Yes, one thing I learned during the study of life events associated with the onset of illness is that patients are eager to discuss their life events, and structuring the content and asking specific questions about different types of life events that may have occurred and when they occurred helps the interviews. This subsequently has implications for the further course of the illness.

It is often the case that the dissemination of research results is influenced by both the initial demand for research and whether the results disappoint or excite the participants. If large segments of society love to drink alcohol, research results that show that consuming alcoholic beverages is harmless or even beneficial are often favored. When it comes to occupational health research, the parties involved tend to emphasize the importance of different research findings. If an employer believes that an organizational restructuring based on the results of an occupational health survey would threaten profitability, managers generally argue against its implementation, while the reverse holds for the labor union. Throughout my career, I have experienced multiple instances where the results were not embraced.

What happens when disagreeable results turn up?

An example illustrating how perceptions of a project can change over time is the experience shared by Annika Härenstam during her doctoral work. She later became a professor of work psychology in Gothenburg. Her dissertation was based on 2000 employees at 67 Swedish correctional facilities. The Director-General of the Swedish Prison and Probation Service at the time was very supportive in the initial stages of the project and generously allowed the research to proceed. However, in the final phase, he became angry and referred to the compiled texts as "that pamphlet." It was unclear to us what had upset him, but one theory was that we had used a blood test that is sensitive to high alcohol consumption (gamma-glutamyl transferase, gamma-GT). It turned out that high levels of this blood marker were more common among the organization's managers, and the effects of poor working conditions on the classic stress hormone cortisol were primarily observed when the gamma-GT levels were high (Härenstam and Theorell, 1990). This suggested that high alcohol consumption could have been a problem in certain groups within the organization. This example can be seen as a general observation. An employer who discovers that the results of an occupational health survey could lead to changes and require significant effort may feel threatened. In this case, it was in addition particularly "hot" to discuss alcohol consumption with the managers who might have had alcohol problems themselves. If the results go against what we desire, we all try to find arguments against them. Sometimes this takes the form of attempting to "poke holes" in the results, even when the research has been well conducted and the findings are well-founded.

C.4 On the Supervisor Role

How is the research student supervised during the PhD process in applied science and, more specifically, in psychosomatic and arts/health fields? This is, of course, an important question for the credibility of applied science since the reputation and trust in these fields depend upon the skills, attitudes, and honesty of those who supervise the production of research results. I have supervised 47 doctoral students on their PhD dissertations during the years 1980–2020. This has given me some insight. There have been many changes in routines for PhD studies during those 40 years. Such changes have pertained to recruitment, how the studies are financed, how their work is supported, and how the formal requirements for the doctoral thesis itself are formulated. Finally, the prospects for the continuation of research activities after obtaining a PhD have changed. During those years I have also seen how the research education has changed since I have participated as a member in numerous dissertation committees and served as opponent in more than forty dissertations not only in Stockholm but also in Uppsala, Umeå, Göteborg, Örebro, Lund/Malmö, Linköping, Bergen, Helsingfors, Oslo, Copenhagen, Aarhus, Aalborg, Oxford, Ghent, Maastricht and Paris.

Despite all the changes in general conditions along with conditions for recruitment, I have always regarded this part of higher education, PhD education, as beneficial for individuals and for society in general. I believe in the value of sharing scientific thinking. I have the same impression from those who teach PhD students in other countries. The PhD programs sharpen the students' analytical ability and increase curiosity among those who pass them. A deeper goal of scientific education is to facilitate the students' ability to take objective critique constructively and to separate objective arguments from personal. This is the most difficult task: to achieve the skill to take objective critique without getting angry. This also pertains to delivering critique, to avoid insulting arguments directed at the person himself/herself. This deeper task is more difficult to attain than other tasks! The supervisor is not always successful in this. But there is mostly a pre-post difference: During the process, the PhD students do become more skilled in separating arguments from the individuals making them.

Why is this important to the general theme of this book? A research career mostly starts with the PhD process. If this functions in an optimal way, the young researcher will have judgment. How do I communicate with society about my research findings? What do I say to journalists if I want to avoid exaggeration but also communicate that the findings may become important if others can replicate them? A functioning PhD learning process will effectively communicate such skills. This is even one of the decisive factors in the building of a reliable image of the role of applied science.

C.5 The Doctoral Student's Own Idea or the Program of the Research Team

Forty out of 47 (85%) of my doctoral students themselves introduced the subject they wanted to focus on in their doctoral thesis. Mostly, the idea evolved during clinical work with patients. Then they turned to me to be their supervisor. In all these thesis production processes, there was a close collaboration in which I could offer ideas about experimental designs and statistical computations, as well as formulations and interpretations. This type of recruitment procedure is not so common today since there are strict rules regarding the financing of projects. In practice, this means that a research group that recruits a new member will aid this person in formulating research applications. It also means that it could be difficult to introduce research ideas that are entirely new for the research group.

The researcher's education has successively become more formalized, which means that it is difficult to combine a researcher education process with clinical work. Researcher education takes place within the framework of a four-year program with strict formal structures. The student receives a grant with a time frame of four years. Within that period, the doctoral thesis shall be produced. One of the difficulties is that a research project may turn out to have unpredictable time delays due to unforeseen obstacles, for instance, difficulties in recruiting participants. All of these external rigid conditions have had the consequence that doctoral students have a lower mean age than they had sixty years ago. The time frame of four years of full-time work can be changed to an individual program lasting for eight years, but it only requires 20 hours of research per week. But most of the students have to accept a full-time schedule lasting for four years. This makes it difficult to stop and start a new program if the real problem is that it is too difficult to recruit a sufficient number of patients or that the research idea turned out to be bad. The lack of flexibility is fertile ground for nervous tension in research students.

For several decades, women have been disfavored in science. Women have had a disadvantage compared to men in winning competitions for grants, which are necessary for starting a research career. This has been important for my doctoral students since the majority are women. Christina Wennerås and Agnes Wold (1997) in Gothenburg made a systematic study of the factors that had statistical significance in determining the likelihood of winning a grant competition. A significant finding was that women had a lower likelihood than men of winning grants in the governmental medical research council when other possible and relevant confounders had been considered.

Another gender-related discussion at the time was the fact that hospitals, for the most part, used male standards for judging whether a patient had a "normal" laboratory test. One of my doctoral students belonged to those researchers who criticized the use of male lab standards. Because of that, she almost lost a competition for a professor position. But she complained to a national reference committee and was finally declared the winner of the competition, against the committee that was assigned to make the judgment! This is very uncommon in these types of processes.

C.6 Inside the Research Community: Might Researchers Themselves Have Destroyed Some of Their Own Credibility: Faking, Exaggerating, Publishing Too Early, and Stealing

In Sweden, we live in an open society with a free press. This means that many conflicts between scientists are described in newspapers. If the discussions are inflammatory, there may be initial efforts to conceal them, but sooner or later, they explode in the mass media. One recent example in Sweden (Vogel, 2023) is the conflicts surrounding Paolo Macchiarini, who was employed in 2010 as a professor of regenerative surgery at the Karolinska Institutet and Hospital. Macchiarini had been performing surgery at first with transplanted throats (trachea) and then with replacement of damaged throats with plastic throats that had been immersed in solutions of cells that should start growing on the plastic surface of these replacement throats. His efforts had been published in highly prestigious scientific journals (among them the Lancet) so he managed to convince the director of the Karolinska Institutet about the groundbreaking future of his activity. However, when he had performed this kind of surgery on one patient in Stockholm in 2011, it turned out that this patient's condition was much worse than it was according to the published article about the case. In 2014, he was reported to the leadership of the Karolinska Institutet for having falsified the results in the Lancet article. All three patients who were operated on in Sweden died, and a long series of difficult processes followed, at first within the scientific community and then in the courts. The leadership of the Karolinska Institutet defended Macchiarini, and serious conflicts arose between defending and accusing colleagues. He was recently convicted (2023) and sentenced to a 2.5-year jail term. It was appealed to the highest court in Sweden, where the verdict was confirmed.

The Macchiarini case illustrates above all that serious problems may arise when the leadership is too protective of its group members. This may hinder correct decisions, and when people in general hear about this, trust in science is adversely affected. It has also been stated that these processes hurt the willingness to take risks in the development of new fields—no experimentally talented surgeon wants to become a new Macchiarini, and more adventurous experiments are avoided, for good or bad. Above all, however, it provides an example of problems within science affecting trust in scientific results. The Macchiarini case falls within the applied science sector since the surgical operations were initiated by faked basic science. If the basic articles had been reported honestly, these operations would not have been made.

Temptations to amplify, manipulate, or even fake research findings are likely to become more prevalent when the degree of competition increases. Competition between research groups has always existed. For instance, in the eighteenth century, was it Carl Wilhelm Scheele or Joseph Priestley who discovered oxygen? (Severinghouse, 2016). Scheele is likely to have discovered it in 1773, but Priestley made the same discovery independently of Scheele in 1774 and was the first one to publish that finding. But another researcher, Michael Sendivogius, may have discovered it even before 1604. More recently, there was an open competition between four different groups of basic scientists to reveal the structure of DNA. However, in the end, the four groups collaborated, and this accelerated the discovery of DNA structure. In both of these examples, we are talking about a healthy and functional competition that could result in collaboration. When we talk about faked or amplified results, the goal is to gain selfish advantage for an individual or a group of researchers at the expense of others—concerning funding, employment, or promotion. At the beginning of my career, faked or manipulated results were very uncommon. With a stronger and stronger "fight for survival," which we see in the science field today, manipulation and dishonesty have become more frequent in the whole world. In applied science, the examples may not be so dramatic as in basic science, and they may play out in more subtle ways. For instance, when a hypothesis (founded in basic science) is tested, for instance, that a particular medication or an environmental intervention has a beneficial effect, the hypothesis testing should follow very strict statistical rules. If many statistical tests are performed at the same time, this must be openly presented and the consequences thereof discussed or statistically handled. A subtle manipulation is to avoid mentioning the number of tests altogether. This can lead to an unwarranted acceptance of positive results. In the scientific discussion, the most important ingredient is total honesty about a study's weaknesses and strengths. During recent years, serious scientific journals have also required a description of donors or supporters of studies. The rationale behind this is, of course, that possible bias should be revealed.

One of my main arguments in this book is that applied science should be used more extensively in societal debates and decision-making. I would add that it should be used not only more extensively but also more wisely. One example of a dubious use of applied science is from the aftermath of the presidential election in the United States in 2020. A large group of voters for the Republican party (and for Donald Trump) became convinced that the election results had been manipulated and that Trump should have won (Ortega, 2020). Epidemiological statistics showed how different counties in Arizona "should" have voted given the distributions of socioeconomic status, race, gender, and age. Given these facts, the proportion of Trump voters was much lower than expected. Thus, the general feeling—that the election was faked—was amplified. However, nothing prevents voters in the "wrong" demographic group from voting outside demographic expectations—in this case, for Joe Biden and not for Donald Trump. In this case, a thorough and active epidemiological discussion using applied science principles could have improved the debate about a "faked" election. Scientists may have contributed to fake processes by not activating normal scientific debates. Neglect to use applied science actively for solving this kind of conflict may, in the long term, undermine trust in it.

Successful scientists are also exposed to temptations to become *gurus*. I am referring to the fact that famous scientists are participating in many newspaper interviews and are expected to have opinions about everything, regardless of whether they have any specific expertise in the subject they are interviewed about. This would be adequate if there were honest statements about the limits of their specific knowledge in the field, but when the scientists start abandoning such principles, this can be problematic. Perhaps the main task of the true scientist is not to offer solutions, but to explain findings and expose limitations—to educate about scientific procedures rather than pretend that they have the final solution.

References

De Manzano, Ö., & Ullén, F. (2018). Same genes, different brains: Neuroanatomical differences between monozygotic twins discordant for musical training. *Cerebral Cortex, 28*(1), 387–394. https://doi.org/10.1093/cercor/bhx299

Demerouti, E., Bakker, A. B., Nachreiner, F., & Schaufeli, W. B. (2001 Jun). The job demands-resources model of burnout. *The Journal of Applied Psychology, 86*(3), 499–512.

Härenstam, A., & Theorell, T. (1990). Cortisol elevation and serum gamma-glutamyl transpeptidase in response to adverse job conditions: How are they interrelated? *Biological Psychology, 31*(2), 157–171. https://doi.org/10.1016/0301-0511(90)90015-o. PMID: 1983313.

Karasek, R. A. (1979). Job demands, job decision latitude, and mental strain: Implications for job redesign. *Administrative Science Quarterly, 1979*, 285–308.

Karasek, R. A., & Theorell, T. (1990). *Healthy work. Stress, productivity and the reconstruction of working life*. Basic Books.

Lennartsson, A.-K., Bojner Horwitz, E., Theorell, T., & Ullén, F. (2017). Creative artistic achievement is related to lower levels of alexithymia. *Creativity Research Journal, 29*(1), 29. https://doi.org/10.1080/10400419.2017.1263507

Lindblad, F., Hogmark, Å., & Theorell, T. (2007). Music intervention for 5th and 6th graders – Effects on development and cortisol secretion. *Stress and Health, 23*, 9–14.

Ortega, B. (2020, December 19). *Arizona republicans worry party infighting could harm them in future elections*. CNN Politics.

Severinghouse, J. W. (2016). Eight sages over five centuries share oxygen's discovery. *Advances in Physiological Education, 40*(3), 370–376. https://doi.org/10.1152/advan.00076.2016

Siegrist, J. (1996). Adverse health effects of high effort/low reward conditions. *Journal of Occupational Health Psychology*, 1, 27–41. https://doi.org/10.1037/1076-8998.1.1.27

Theorell, T. (2009). Anabolism and catabolism. In S. Sonnentag, P. L. Perrewé, & D. S. Ganster (Eds.), *Research in occupational stress and wellbeing. Current perspectives on job-stress recovery* (Vol. 7, pp. 249–276). Emerald Group.

Theorell, T. (2020). The demand control support work stress model. In T. Theorell (Ed.), *Handbook of socioeconomic determinants of occupational health. From macro-level to micro-level evidence*. Springer Reference Books.

Theorell, T. (2022). Psychosocial stressors in psychosomatic cardiology: A narrative review. *Heart and Mind, 6*, 211–218. https://doi.org/10.4103/hm.hm_26_22

Theorell, T. (2023). *Psychosocial risk factors at work and mental ill health*. OSH Wiki. European Agency for Safety and Health at work. Published on: 25/07/2023. Latest update: 25/07/2023.

Theorell, T., Lind, E., Fröberg, J., Karlsson, C. G., & Levi, L. (1972 Nov–Dec). A longitudinal study of 21 subjects with coronary heart disease: Life changes, catecholamine excretion and related biochemical reactions. *Psychosomatic Medicine, 34*(6), 505–516. https://doi.org/10.1097/00006842-197211000-00003

Theorell, T., Lennartsson, A.-K., Mosing, M. A., & Ullén, F. (2014). Musical activity and emotional competence – A twin study. *Frontiers in Psychology, 16*(5), 774.

Theorell, T., De Manzano, Ö., Lennartsson, A. K., Pedersen, N. L., & Ullén, F. (2016). Self-reported psychological demands, skill discretion and decision authority at work: A twin study. *Scandinavian Journal of Public Health, 44*(4), 354–360. https://doi.org/10.1177/1403494815626610. Epub 2016 Jan 29. PMID: 26825630.

Vogel, G. (2023). Disgraced surgeon Paolo Macchiarini, whose crimes inspired an opera, headed to prison. *Science*. https://doi.org/10.1126/science.zzrxjtp

Weber, E. W., Spychiger, M., & Patry, J.-L. (1993). *Musik macht Schule: Biografie und Ergebnisse eines Schulversuchs mit erweitertem Musikunterricht* (Pädagogik in der Blauen Eule) (Vol. 17). Die Blaue Eule.

Wennerås, C. and Wold, A. (1997). Nepotism and sexism in peer-review. *Nature*, 387, 341-343. https://doi.org/10.1038/387341a0

Communication with Society

D.1 To What Extent Do People Trust Results from Different Kinds of Science?

When we approach the question of whether people in general believe in science or not, one could speculate that people's trust in science, to some extent, reflects the trust the scientists have for one another within science. Figure 1 in the introductory Chap. "Introduction: Why Do People Not Listen?" illustrates that a general feeling of distrust between scientists is contagious in the sense that malicious and negative judgments regarding other researchers' scientific activities, particularly when communicated to newspapers and social media, are likely to decrease society's trust in science in general. On the other hand, if scientists maintain a respectful way of communicating, even when they disagree about the interpretation of results, it is likely to contribute to trust.

In Sweden, as in the United States and many other countries, we have scientific institutions that examine political opinions by using surveys, for instance, the likelihood that you would vote for the Republicans or the Democrats. But they could also be about trust that people feel in different kinds of societal institutions. Such surveys may also include questions about people's confidence in scientific institutions. This has been going on since 2002 in Sweden.

Figure 1 (in this chapter) shows the percentage of participants in the surveys conducted by the SOM Institute at Gothenburg University. Respondents are assumed to represent the Swedish total adult population. The number of invited subjects varied between 6000 (2002) and 24,000 (2020), and the participation rate was between 60% (2002) and 48% (2020). Weighting for particularly low participation in certain groups has been performed. The numbers in the y axis indicate the percentage who reported "very good" or "rather good" trust in medical (green) and societal (blue) scientific results, respectively. The numbers under the x axis indicate the years from 2002 to 2020.

© The Author(s), under exclusive license to Springer Nature
Switzerland AG 2025
T. Theorell, *Underuse of Applied Science in Changing Societies*, SpringerBriefs
in Public Health, https://doi.org/10.1007/978-3-031-96391-9_5

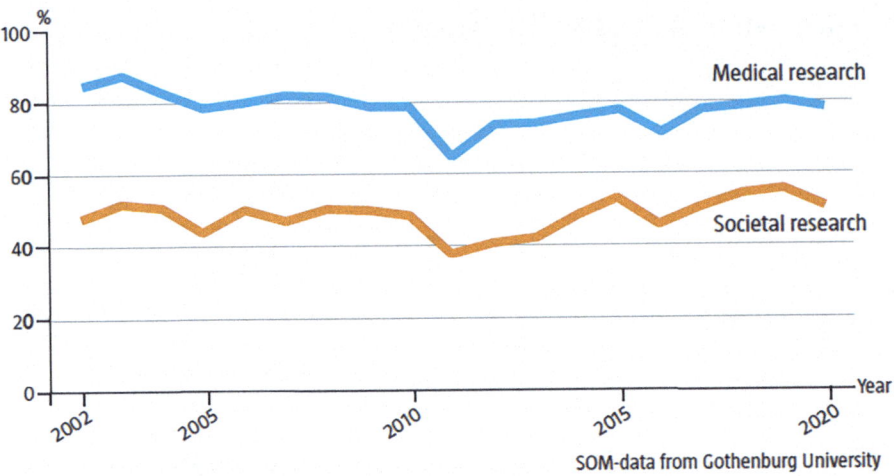

Fig. 1 Trust in medical and societal research in Sweden, 2002–2020. (Source: SOM Institute, Gothenburg University; Credit: Annika Röhl, 2025)

According to the results, confidence in medical science has been constantly high during the 2000s. Between 77% and 85% of the people who responded to this survey said that they trusted medical science. The figure does not cover the pandemic years, but during that period, trust in medical science even increased slightly. In addition, participants trust technological science. Seventy percent have confidence in that. Natural science is also a discipline that people have regarded with high confidence, but that has decreased in later years, down to 60%. For social science, however, confidence is much lower, between 45% and 50%. For research in education and humanistic subjects, the confidence is quite low, between 35% and 50%.

Figure 1 shows trust in medical and societal research among Swedes between 2002 and 2020. The numbers for humanistic research are very similar to those for societal research.

The source of this information is the SOM (Society, Opinion and Media) Institute (2023).

For the kind of research that I have been doing, which occupies a position between medical science and educational science, it could be expected to be 60%. People could say, "Oh, that's fine, 60% confidence in what you say when you make a statement in the newspaper." But, unfortunately, the other side of this is also true, which means that 40% of people reading that newspaper article will have no confidence in the statement I am making. This mirrors, in a nutshell, a serious problem that faces today's applied science.

The most recent results (Johansson Palmqvist et al., 2024) from the continuous monitoring of research shows that confidence in research continues to be high (86% respond that they feel confidence in university researchers), but a striking finding is that in the youngest group included in these surveys (age 16–29), confidence in research has decreased substantially from 81% to 66%. A possible positive interpretation of this could be that pupils in high school are taught to be critical of information, but it could also mirror a growing feeling of distrust in science among young people. Another new trend is that more participants in the science survey are pessimistic regarding the technical development. Thus, one in five participants (22%) believe that modern technical development will make life worse. This has been a dramatic change since the year 2022, when this question was also asked of the participants, and only 8% believed that technical development could make life worse. This is probably mirroring the recent discussion regarding artificial intelligence.

I have been doing a substantial amount of research on conditions in the workplace. And we encounter this lack of societal trust all the time. If you want to prohibit things or say that conditions in the work environment are so dangerous that people are dying, then employers are more likely to dislike our results. However, unions are likely to embrace them.

One of our research projects was on employees in prisons and their work environment. There were hundreds of prisons included in this study. The general director of our Swedish prisons was all for it. He was very friendly and supported us. But then, when the results came out, they indicated that bosses in prisons were perhaps drinking too much alcohol. This was associated with increased work environment problems in the prisons. Suddenly, the general director of Swedish prisons disliked our research and regarded it as a bad pamphlet.

So, in the moment when the research results become unpleasant for the management, they are less likely to be supported by the management itself.

Politicians and the public interpret what they read in their own way. For instance, if people love to drink alcohol, they like research reports that say alcohol is good for you. But if you think that alcohol should be prohibited in society, then you only like the articles that agree.

When researchers working with applied science are interviewed in newspapers and other mass media, they are frequently tempted to make rather simple and monolithic statements, such as, "According to our research, these kinds of particles in the air cause lung cancer." However, in the head of the researcher, this statement is surrounded by circumstantial conditions that may increase or decrease this particular risk. In addition, the subjects examined may have been exclusively female or only working in white-collar jobs. Therefore, the findings cannot be generalized. All these conditions are in the researcher's mind but are lost to the readers of the resulting text. The interview situation, and even more so the space that the journalist has for summarizing the presented results, do not allow for a more detailed description of such conditions. The most important background factor is, of course, how the researchers arrived at the specific conclusion. How many participants were included? Is that number sufficient for statistical calculations? How were the participants approached—by advertisements, employee lists, or among friends? Do the partici-pants really represent a defined group, for instance, the Swedish population? How reliable are the assessments themselves? Are there financial interests behind the study? It is perhaps not surprising that the credibility of applied science suffers when, again and again, it happens that a particular result later turns out to be wrong or misleading. Unfortunately, news media favors brief and "brand new" findings, and when society has become aware of the "hottest" research news, the likelihood that the responsible researcher will be funded for future efforts increases. In some good universities, researchers are trained in communication with the mass media. The researcher may be taught in such courses not to publish results before the whole scientific within-group discussion has made the findings as scrutinized as possible. That is already hard since there may be competition with other research groups, and being first is important. It is also difficult for the simple reason that discoveries are perceived as particularly important.

It is possible that trust in applied science would improve if knowledge in the population regarding the scientific processing of studies and results could be improved. That would perhaps also decrease the likelihood that political arguments like "scientists constitute an interest group, their arguments should not weigh more heavily than those of other interest groups" are used in societal debates. The average citizen is not aware of the nature of scientific data collection and analysis, and that the whole idea of scientific endeavors is to make efforts to disregard external inter-ests. Complaints about scientists and their "ivory towers" and their formulations made on "writing desks without input from the real world" are prevalent. But the reverse is mostly true: The scientific data collected are based upon what ordinary people say, concentrations of good or bad agents in their bodies, and visits to hospi-tals or deaths. The researchers summarize such data from real people in the popula-tion in a systematic way.

Another aspect of the growing distrust in applied science is that the willingness to participate in population-based studies has decreased. In the Scandinavian coun-tries, there has traditionally been a high participation rate in population studies. Statistics Sweden has had the responsibility for data collection regarding various aspects of health and wellness, social networks, work environment, and financial situation. From 1968, several such *cohort* studies were started. They were based on randomly selected citizens, either in face-to-face or telephone interviews. Participation rates in the order of 80–90% were obtained. During later years, the participation rates have decreased substantially and are now mostly in the order of 50%. When population studies with such low participation rates are performed, doubts about their representativeness are inevitable. There are many potential rea-sons for this decrease. One is, for instance, that population surveys have become increasingly popular in non-scientific fields. Companies often want to announce that their products are popular, and therefore, they send out questionnaires explor-ing the attitudes towards the product.

In summary, trust in applied science is not as widespread as often assumed, and this is, of course, a major problem in communication between applied scientists and the surrounding society.

D.2 Fight Between Different Kinds of Research Methods and Points of View: Examples from Psychosomatic Research on Clinical Practices—Intellectual Fights Are Necessary in Applied Science

That social medicine, stress, and psychosomatic medicine were not regarded as important subjects for those with the most influence in medical research was something I had understood early in my career. Even though Stewart Wolf was world famous and regarded as a big star during a series of international congresses—Society, Stress, and Disease—in Stockholm during the 1960s and 1970s. I understood when I worked with Wolf at the University of Texas (1972–1973) that these subjects were not regarded as important among mainstream medical researchers in the corridors of his university. They talked with indulgence about this "soft" research (which I did not regard as soft at all). Lennart Levi himself was a controversial figure among medical researchers in Sweden. I have had such experiences myself. I started my career after finishing my physician education, working both clinically and with research in cardiology (although my interest in psychosomatic medicine was used in my doctoral thesis work). After 11 years, I decided to move to social medicine, which was in a large, newly built hospital. It clearly illustrated to me that cardiology had a much higher position than social medicine. When I met colleagues in the corridors and they asked where I worked in the hospital, they looked frightened and almost pitied me when I mentioned social medicine.

During the 1970s to 1990s, there was an intense fight between "psychodynamic" and "biological" perspectives in psychological science. This fight is still ongoing. I belonged to those who tried to initiate a constructive dialogue between the two antagonistic schools. During my time as chairman of the Society for Medical Psychology (which belonged to the Swedish Association of Physicians), I tried to organize a program with both psychodynamic and biological themes. However, it turned out to be impossible to initiate a dialogue—the *biologists* came only when the lecturer had a known *biological* name and vice versa.

The debate between psychodynamic and biological interpretations is activated now and then. Ten years ago, it restarted during the debates regarding a patient who was in forced care (the Säter case, Råstam, 2017) in a department of forensic psychiatry. I am not in a position to interpret all the evidence, but he was accused of having committed several murders. In later stages of the long-lasting law processes, he was acquitted, and the question was: How could the law process end up drawing such erroneous conclusions? One of the main problems was that the police officers responsible for the criminal technical examinations were so impressed by new theories regarding memory retention that they disregarded their forensic findings and did not pursue their possible clues to persons who may have committed the respective murders. A similar problem arose because principles used in psycho-dynamically oriented treatment were mixed up with evidence used in criminal examinations. To be more specific, a specific memory of an event described by a patient may be very useful in a therapeutic process, despite not being necessarily true from a criminal technical point of view. Mixing therapy and criminal examination could be quite dangerous when the therapeutic memory is not supported by criminal technological examinations. Unfortunately, this creates a situation in which all psychodynamic therapeutic principles are regarded with suspicion (Josefsson, 2013). I have been supervising several students who believe in psychodynamically influenced theories, and I believe that such theories are of value in the interpretation of the interplay between people and therapeutic principles. But they are mostly useless in criminal examinations.

Psychodynamic theories should not be mixed up with qualitative research. Qualitative research could start with individual descriptions of events surrounding the onset of an illness, environmental changes, subjective experiences during the final stages of a dying process, or anything. The important goal is to arrive at a full description of an important event (or series of events) in the eyes of the central person. Statistical aspects are not relevant. Qualitative and statistical descriptions supplement each other in a major research endeavor. Many of the doctoral theses that I have supervised have contained both quantitative and qualitative aspects. In general, this has been unproblematic, but on a few occasions, conflicts have arisen. The worst conflict concerned (Elander Lindberg, 1997) the work of a clinically active psychologist who had treated patients with rheumatoid arthritis. She had produced careful notes after each clinical consultation. She collaborated with her husband, who was a rheumatologist. In the protocols, it was possible to follow both results from blood analyses (mainly a test showing the activity of the rheumatoid process) and from psychological discussions and descriptions of ongoing life events and emotional states. The plan was to recruit independent clinicians who could be instructed to grade various medical and psychological dimensions from the consultations and blood tests. With the use of statistics, this would have created a unique possibility to throw light on the interrelationships between psychological and immunological processes in rheumatoid arthritis.

Unfortunately, we were unable to recruit an independent researcher judge for the assessments, but the doctoral student asked her husband to do the assessments. Since he could be regarded as biased and, in addition, had a background of clinical responsibility for some of the medical treatments, his assessments could not be regarded as independent or unbiased. This was the most difficult problem. However, in addition, one other part of the doctoral thesis treated another group of patients, namely those with symptoms of *oral galvanism*. Oral galvanism was a highly debated disease at the time. A patient pressure group was arguing that the symptoms typical of galvanism were due to mercury seals in their teeth. The argument was that the seals were leaking mercury into the blood of the patients and that this explained their symptoms, which were all of a general nature, such as fatigue and diffuse pain. My doctoral student argued that such symptoms could also be explained in psychological terms, and her patient's notations were used as arguments. However, her arguments were hard to verify, and counterarguments were formulated by the patient groups and their physicians and dentists. The patients themselves disliked the thought that their symptoms were not due to their mercury seals.

There were five members of the examination committee. The usual number of members on such a committee was three, but when the subject was transdisciplinary, the number of committee members was extended to five. The members were always asked in advance whether or not the thesis could be used in a doctoral dissertation. In this case, the recommendation was: "Do not arrange a dissertation!" I was asked to tell the doctoral student about this non-recommendation, which I did—"Do not defend your thesis!" But she used her right protected in Swedish law to defend her thesis. The dissertation lasted for eight hours, starting at 1 pm. Several opposing statements were not announced in advance. The examination committee used two hours for discussions regarding the decision (pass or fail). The whole procedure accordingly lasted for ten hours and was finished at 11 pm. The thesis passed (three members for and two against).

The atmosphere around this doctoral thesis was unusually inflammatory. Part of this was due to the psychosomatic nature of the studied relationships. However, immunological research has already been published that supports the idea that critical life changes and psychologically poor living conditions may have adverse effects on the clinical course of rheumatoid arthritis. Epidemiological research has subsequently been published from the Karolinska Institutet showing that stressful conditions at work can trigger the onset of rheumatoid arthritis (Bengtsson et al., 2009). However, when a shift in paradigms is under way the scientific arguments must be clear and verifiable. The specialist in rheumatology in the committee elegantly formulated this: "Science should be the most democratic activity in science. Outsiders should be able to read and understand what has been done and it should be possible for outsiders to redo the same experiment." We had failed to find independent people willing to do the independent ratings, verifying or not verifying the conclusions made by the authors. Accordingly, this thesis was a shaky product. However, the system is constructed mainly for the protection of doctoral students. It is really hard to make a thesis "non-passing." That requires the discovery of faked findings or plagiarism in the text. Neither of those could be applied in this particular case.

The intensive discussions regarding this thesis about psychosomatic mechanisms accelerated discussions about the introduction of a compulsory statement by the examination committee, written before the dissertation—a statement issued at least three weeks before the public event recommending the dissertation. All the members of the committee should have examined the quality of the proposed thesis before printing. This change was instituted in all the medical faculties in our country.

At the beginning of my research studies, registered nurses were not allowed to start research education (since their clinical education is much shorter than the medical education), unless they had finished some other clinical education, for instance, as a psychologist. During the 1980s, such a possibility was created for this group. If they supplemented their clinical nurse education with academic points, for instance in psychology, biochemistry, or physiology, according to an individualized plan, they could be allowed to start a researcher education. This development has been described by Hamrin et al. (2014).

The first nurses who went all the way to doctoral dissertations were regarded with great suspicion by many medical researchers. The first obstetric nurse who defended a PhD thesis in the Nordic countries was Vivianne Wahlberg (1982), whose thesis was about Credé prophylaxis, which was a routine introduced in 1881. The Credé prophylaxis aimed at the prevention of gonococcal eye infection in the newborn. It was an important procedure—by dripping drops of silver nitrate in the eyes of the newborn, this serious eye infection could be prevented. If the mother suffered from gonococcal infection, this could be directly transferred to the newborn, and blindness was a common consequence of gonorrhoeic eye infection. In 1881, there were no antibiotic treatments available for this. When Vivianne Wahlberg defended her doctoral thesis a hundred years after the introduction of the Credé prophylaxis, however, there were several antibiotic treatments available against gonorrhoeic infections. And dripping silver nitrate into the eyes of the newborn was not without complications, since this chemical compound causes a strong irritation in the eyes. Systematic observations of a series of newborns during the first days after delivery by Vivianne Wahlberg showed that the eyes of the newborn were closed during that period, which was not the case in a comparable group of infants who had not been subjected to the Credé prophylaxis. This means that the possibility for the newborn to establish contact with the mother during the first period after birth was seriously inhibited.

During the dissertation, it became evident that the importance of the lost eye contact between newborn and mother was judged differently by different groups of caregivers surrounding the newborn. The microbiologists and ophthalmologists worried more about the infection itself than about the mother-child contact. They worried about the risk that the gonorrhoeic infection might be diagnosed too late without the Credé prophylaxis. The pediatricians, obstetricians, and obstetric nurses, on the other hand, rated the hampered mother-child contact as more important than bacteriological risks. However, the dissertation and the discussions that followed led to the decision to abandon the Credé prophylaxis in obstetrics! This conclusion resulted in the abandonment of the Credé prophylaxis in obstetrical units in all of Sweden.

This discussion represents an interesting example in applied science. It weighs a "soft" risk (inhibited mother-child contact) against a "hard" risk (infection and blindness). It also represents a science development discussion—when is it right to abandon an established prevention routine? This example furthermore shows that sometimes applied science can indeed serve as a useful judging process in a societal situation with differing opinions, and the objective observations of the newborn babies were an important ingredient in the final decision.

One of my doctoral nursing students, Caroline Häggmark, had a very concrete question in her thesis work. She worked with cancer care and the question could be formulated in the following way: If relatives of cancer patients are allowed to spend more time with the patient in the ward and if these relatives learn more about practical care, including how to make injections and feed the patient, will that make them more willing to offer home care for the patient, with support from staff? Accordingly, the relatives of one group of patients were offered such possibilities, and another group, or relatives of a similar group of cancer patients, served as the comparison group. Observations were made before and at the end of the intervention/control period. Two-thirds of the patients died (in both groups) during the study. Contrary to expectations, the relatives who had participated more actively in the care of the patients were much more unwilling to take the patients home for home care than the relatives in the control group. This is probably explained by the increased awareness of all the difficulties that caring relatives will face as home carers. Another important observation was that during the final phase preceding the patient's death, the plasma cortisol levels were significantly elevated in the intervention group but not in the control group relatives. One month and two months *before* the death of the patient, the plasma cortisol levels were elevated in the *intervention relatives*, but not in the relatives, in the control group. On the other hand, at examination one and two months *after* the death of the patient, the questionnaire scores for mental exhaustion were significantly *lower* in the intervention group relatives than in the control group relatives. This is consistent with the idea that grief was activated (with cortisol elevation) by the active participation in the care, but also with the idea that activated mourning may have prophylactic value for the relatives after the patient's death.

The findings were unexpected: The relatives who participated more in the care of the patient were less willing than the relatives in the other group to take the patient to home care (Häggmark, 1990). The politicians in the county responsible for the cancer care had donated money to the project because they hoped this could reduce the length of the hospital care period (and save money for the county). The other unexpected finding was that relatives in the group with active care participation showed more physiological (increased cortisol) and psychological distress during the terminal phase of the patient's illness, but on the other hand this turned out to be beneficial for them after the death of the patient (Theorell et al., 1987).

It may be symptomatic that the only doctoral thesis that did not pass during the long period when I worked as a researcher at the Karolinska Institutet was indeed defended by an obstetric nurse. The obstetric nurses are doing very concrete work, and the recommendations resulting from their scientific work are therefore likely to result in very practical discussions. The thesis that did not pass was addressing the following question: "Do the 'pain killing' routines in obstetric care influence the babies as adult persons?"

All deliveries that took place in one of the regional obstetric clinics in the Stockholm area (at the time there were very few home deliveries and deliveries in private institutions) during the years 1945 to 1966 were followed up, and the "babies" were 20 to 40 years old at the time of the follow-up.

The results (Jacobson et al., 1990) showed that there was indeed a relationship between pain management and mortality later in adult age among the newborns. If the mother had received high dosages of nitrogen oxide ("laughing gas") during the delivery, there was a future elevated risk in the infant to develop dependency on amphetamine-like drugs in adult years. Similarly, high dosages of pethidine (a morphine-like pain killer) to the mother turned out to be correlated with an elevated risk in the newborn in future adult years to develop dependency on morphine-like drugs. Those results passed the examination, but there was also an article dealing with babies who had their umbilical cord around their neck. In these cases, the future adults turned out to have an elevated risk of suicide in the form of hanging during the follow-up years. The proposed theory was that these babies had developed a choking sensation, which led them to commit suicide using that method. That interpretation was judged as too speculative by the committee, and therefore, the thesis did not pass. But the doctoral student came back with a new version, which did not include the most controversial article, at which point the thesis did pass.

It is possible that all three outcomes that were discussed had one common denominator: that this area of Stockholm during that period was an area with many drug addicts and psychiatrically ill people. When the children grew up in such families, they may have seen drug addict behaviors, which may have influenced their risk of illness. In addition, if their mothers during their pregnancies had been disturbed and frequently agitated and nervous, this may have increased the risk that the baby swirled around in the uterus more frequently than other babies, which increased the risk of the umbilical cord wrapping around the neck. In other words, these children grew up in psychiatrically ill conditions, and that may be the underlying cause of the observed correlations. Regardless of interpretation, the observations were valuable. They pointed out strong reasons for public health work in the area.

The parallels between the Credé prophylaxis and the long-term correlations between pain killing during delivery and serious morbidity in the baby as an adult are obvious. The findings had very concrete potential implications for delivery practice, and in both cases, nurses were the defendants during the dissertation. The study of relatives in cancer care also had strong practical implications, but since the findings did not indicate any potential financial gain in introducing expanded participation of relatives in cancer care, this thesis did not cause intense discussions. The psychosomatic rheumatological examination caused intense discussion, but this was mainly due to conflicts in the scientific community between different schools of thinking.

There is no doubt that the rapid introduction and growth of nursing research (performed by registered nurses) introduced new important perspectives in health care. The first decades in nursing research in Sweden have been described in an anthology (Hamrin et al., 2014). Unfortunately, nursing research applications have not received the attention that they deserve, so this is one obvious example of applied research that is not sufficiently used in society. In my field, nursing research has been a close ally, which is obvious in the large proportion of nursing researchers among my PhD students.

D.3 From Accepting Relationships Between Psychosocial Conditions and Bodily Changes to Choosing Remedies

Fundamental fights between different schools of thinking are still ongoing, although the fighting ditches may have moved. Today, it is possible to use advanced methods for the study of ongoing thinking processes in different parts of the brain, for instance, using functional magnetic resonance imaging (fMRI). It is also possible to record minute changes in the blood concentration of different hormones. In addition, it has become possible to record minute changes in heart muscle or gut activity. One would expect such fundamental scientific developments to result in the solution of conflicts in scientific thinking. However, that is not happening. The overriding thoughts about human existence are probably the same as they were during the fifteenth century, and it seems to me that some people are not willing to accept the thought that our external social and psychological conditions can influence our psyche in ways that induce bodily changes. It may not matter how many fantastic proofs we present.

Figure 1 from the chapter entitled "How Does Applied Science Operate?" describes the job strain story and shows how the work environment and the individual-psychological domains relate to one another. The work domain directly gives rise to reactions, but it also evokes reactions through the individual program, which is determined partly by the genetic makeup and partly by previous experiences that accumulate throughout life. It should be pointed out that genetic makeup is not working in isolation. A relatively new research field is epigenetics: Genes that determine stress reactions are sensitized by environmental conditions that frequently give rise to frightening conditions. The opposite conditions are also true; in a safe environment, stress genes become desensitized. Some of the chemistry behind such sensitization/desensitization is known—the genes may be methylated or demethylated (Szyf, 2012). Changes in gene sensitivity may occur throughout life, although a substantial part of this sensitivity is established during childhood. Accordingly, it is not sufficient to treat the individual in isolation; one must take the environment into account. The job strain story illustrates the importance of the psychosocial work environment, for instance. By reorganization and improved leadership, it is possible to prevent and treat sick work environments.

The figure also illustrates another important aspect of the interplay between the individual and the environment in relation to health. This is that the individuals may be aware or unaware of their behavioral reactions—changes in smoking, drinking, and jogging habits, for instance. Somebody may have to increase their awareness of special education programs. This is an important activity in public and occupational health institutions. Subjects may also be aware of or unaware of their psychological reactions, which is an important task for psychological and psychiatric institutions. Those who are unaware of their psychological reactions (as well as of those of others) are labeled *alexithymic*. Finally, body awareness could vary between different groups. As an active physician, I was often stunned by the lack of bodily awareness, so this may also have to be taught, for instance, by means of heart rate or blood pressure monitoring.

Accepting relationships between psychosocial processes and bodily changes is one thing. The next step, even when we talk about the individual part, is to choose individual remedies (when they are needed) in order to decrease illness risk and to treat illness once it has arisen. There are fundamentally different schools of thinking. During later years in Sweden, there has been a fight about the role of cognitive behavioral therapy (CBT) vs. psychodynamic therapy in psychological and psychosomatic illness. Various forms of CBT have indeed been proven in randomized controlled trials to be effective in decreasing symptoms of depression, anxiety, and exhaustion (Öst et al., 2023). But more psychodynamically oriented methods have also been shown to be effective, for instance, in decreasing depression in randomized controlled studies (Caselli et al., 2023). At present, there seems to be no clear evidence for favoring CBT vs. psychodynamic treatment, but the national policy has favored CBT. It could be that CBT effects are more rapid, whereas psychodynamic therapies have more long-lasting effects. Different groups of patients prefer different kinds of therapy. It is important that there are alternatives with proven benefits.

In the discussions surrounding psychosocial factors and their importance to health, the positive vs. negative perspective is also important. The Israeli American sociologist Aaron Antonovsky, during his later career as a researcher, introduced the concept of *salutogenesis*, which refers to factors that stimulate health (Antonovsky, 1979). They are the sociological counterpart of the regeneration concept that is used in physiology. He was striking an important chord because the concept became very popular among researchers involved in subjects that are relevant to stress and psychosomatic medicine. His focus was originally on conditions that determined health despite major difficulties, for instance, so-called *Dandelion Children* (with a difficult childhood background) and Jewish children who had been kept in concentration camps for a long time. He wanted to find conditions that could explain why individuals who had been living in extremely difficult conditions could later in life lead a healthy life despite the atrocities they had experienced. Antonovsky constructed a questionnaire assessing *Sense of Coherence* (SOC). That has been translated into several languages. There are three components in SOC: comprehensibility, manageability, and meaningfulness. The theory is good for scientific discussions, but the questionnaire does not function so well in practice. One of the dimensions, meaningfulness, is close to depression questionnaires (Henje Blom et al., 2010). When an individual is depressed, everything seems meaningless to him or her. It has been shown that the mean SOC score decreases in the population during periods of high unemployment, like in Sweden during the 1990s (Nilsson et al., 2003). Another problem with the use of scores derived from the SOC questionnaire is that extraordinarily high scores can be found in religious fanatic sects or criminal gangs—such groups tend to isolate themselves socially from the surrounding society. In such a group, a high SOC score reflects the isolation from society and the strong interdependence the members have.

The discussion surrounding the concept of sense of coherence illustrates that psychosomatic studies need simple, easy-to-understand theories, but also that methodological and conceptual problems arise in the application of such theories. Some of it leads to open quarreling between different scientific schools, especially when amplified by the media. This may contribute to the underuse of applied science.

Psychosocial studies of societal conditions have been criticized for overemphasizing negative aspects of working conditions while neglecting positive aspects. While there is certainly some truth in the critique, it is also true that most of the concepts that psychosocial researchers use are graded from the worst to the best conditions. Accordingly, they are not bipolar (either bad or good). Hence, the absence of good conditions is mostly described as low ratings on a psychosocial scale. Finally, the argument that research should put more emphasis on finding *good* conditions may be an excuse for doing nothing about the bad conditions. These discussions are sometimes translated into societal discussions in which political parties may choose one or the other side. This adds further confusion to the debate. In the highly respected American magazine, *The Economist* (Sept 24, 2016), Schumpeter described how some American companies are observing whether individual employees smile sufficiently often, and whether they are communicating enough smiles in their emails. Those employees who produce too few smiles cannot expect a raise in the annual salary negotiation. This is likely to give rise to convoluted joy with underlying tensions. If questions regarding a good work environment are neglected because a considerable amount of energy is consumed by the production of "false joy," we may be on the wrong track. Joy should not be a forced phenomenon, but spontaneous.

D.4 Pros and Cons: Difficulties for Citizens to Assess Messages from Applied Science

Lay people sometimes must make very practical decisions regarding their participation or nonparticipation in societal processes. In these decisions, applied science may be of great importance. One example is the debate regarding participation or nonparticipation in vaccination against COVID-19.

Pro-vaccination: It has been estimated (Meslé et al., 2024) in 34 countries or areas, where it was possible to examine this, that vaccinations reduced mortality by 59% overall, representing 1.6 million lives among those aged 25 years or older during a period of 2.5 years (2020–2023). For instance, those states in the United States that had a low vaccination prevalence had a more pronounced increase in mortality during the COVID pandemic. A high vaccination prevalence in the population, as well as a high protective effect of the vaccine, are required for so-called *herd immunity*, which is the goal in mass vaccination. The argument is that the higher the percentage of the population that has been vaccinated, the lower the risk that the illness will spread. This means that a person who is vaccinated allows this individual not only to have the benefit of a lower individual risk of falling ill, developing serious illness, and even dying, but also contributes to a lowered spread in the population.

Against vaccination: There is a small risk that vaccination may lead to complications. The most serious complication that has been described is sleeping illness, which is very uncommon. The individual who is wondering whether to allow vaccination or not accordingly has to weigh this possible small individual risk of developing vaccine-related serious complications against the much higher benefit of avoiding death both for themselves and to contribute to a lowered risk for the whole population. Unfortunately, citizens are often hindered from finding a balanced debate. Pressure groups with a very unbalanced opinion about the scientific interpretations start trying to make citizens avoid vaccination, even using fake arguments. Active efforts could even be made to hide the facts. It is difficult in that situation, as a lay person, to make good decisions.

An important conclusion that could be drawn is that it is important to teach how applied science functions and what principles guide it:

1. It is about getting as close as possible to the truth, and pointing out complexities which could mean that the best solutions may have to be differentiated.
2. Scientists are not gurus and should not act like gurus, but a scientist involved in each subject can mostly contribute important information and meaningful opinions. Unfortunately, simplicity is seductive, and daily newspapers like scientists who present simple explanations without complicated diversity. In other words, we scientists may enjoy the guru role in which we can gain popularity. We sometimes have to fight ourselves in this.
3. When a new problem arises in society, science needs time for examining it and for making suggestions regarding solutions. Diversity of opinion is normal at the beginning of that process. That scientists quarrel is normal and not evidence of crookedness, as lay people without knowledge about how science functions may suspect when they see headlines about scientific diversity in newspapers.
4. People in general need knowledge about how science functions and how to interpret simple messages in newspapers. Credibility of research results depends on methods for data collection, reliability of assessments, appropriateness of statistical methods, representativeness of study samples, and possible bias among researchers (which should be openly declared if there is any).

However, the vaccination example is also important because it illustrates the tension between egocentric and collective rationales in this kind of individual decision-making. The individual must weigh the minute risk of developing a rare vaccine complication against a possible benefit for the whole population, including himself/herself. The vaccine complication is very concrete and close to the individual, whereas the benefit for the population and a possible decrease in one's own risk are more remote and theoretical.

A societal problem that relates to applied research is the use of witness reports from small children who can easily be manipulated, but whose memories may be powerful tools. New basic science has taught us that early experiences in life influence the development of the structure of our brains (see, for instance, Jeong et al., 2021). Accordingly, on a societal basis, it is necessary to protect children from traumatic experiences because subjects who have had such experiences as children are likely to have less functional brains than others. For instance, according to Jeong et al., their brain cortex is thinner than that of other comparable subjects in the population. But this does not mean that witness reports from small children are necessarily useful in court trials about possible abuse. Such distinctions have to be explained, particularly to police agents and judges who have the responsibility in trials.

Collective processes arising in society may make the choices even more difficult for the individual. A politician who becomes identified with one choice, for instance, against vaccination, starts to build their electability on this identity. If they change their mind, they may lose a large number of voters. Increasingly, they will find it difficult to leave this position even if they become convinced that this has been wrong.

An important discussion relates to the position of fine arts (music, theater, visual arts, including movie production, literature) in society. There is rapidly growing literature which shows that early engagement of small children in music training promotes the development of: (a) finger skills, (b) emotion handling, and to some extent, (c) cognitive development. This is obviously of great potential importance for politicians. Why are they not more interested? First, politicians do not like to favor societal programs that have difficult-to-predict outcomes. An important competitor for societal attention is physical activity. That increased physical activity can improve public health has been extensively proven in multiple studies. Outcomes are relatively predictable on a societal level. It is to some extent possible to provide quantitative predictions. If we increase jogging stimuli, how many organizations and how many employees do we need to achieve a given reduction in the incidence of type 2 diabetes in the population? The effects of cultural activity are more unpredictable. They give energy to the population, but this energy may have unpredictable directions. If politicians distribute increasing amounts of money to theatres, will that give them political benefit? No, not necessarily, the theatres may start producing plays that are critical of current politics. Many of Shakespeare's plays are voices in ongoing political debates at the time. The same statement applies to music, visual arts, and literature. Dictators such as Stalin, Hitler, and Mao Zedong have been fully aware of this problem, and their solution has been to decide what kind of cultural activity they want to stimulate. Other political regimes, such as the Taliban, have prohibited culture in general (Theorell, 2016). But there have also been positive examples in the history of societies that have produced a culture to favor democratic solutions to societal problems. A famous example is the Greek play *The Oresteia* by Aeschylus (458 BC). The aim was to make the Athenians accept the idea that voting as a way of solving societal problems is superior to violence.

All kinds of cultural activities could be regarded as tools for magnifying social and psychological processes. Accordingly, they could not be regarded as per se "good" or "bad." Strong pieces of theater, music, and paintings/sculptures could be used to magnify both evil and good. But a well-organized society should allow its citizens to use cultural activities for the expression of their thoughts.

The unpredictable nature of cultural activities in general is probably one of the reasons why politicians hesitate to take in results from applied research on social, psychological, and biological effects of cultural activities. How much of a role the government should play in providing means to produce theater, music, visual arts, and literature has been a constant subject for discussion ever since organized societies existed. If private donations dominate financial support, there is a risk of commercialization with unpredictable consequences, and vice versa, if the government dominates, there is always a risk that evil politicians can start using culture for domination of opinions. The response to this could be to provide cultural diversity at school so that children become interested in cultural expressions that are not only contemporary and popular but also from other epochs and countries. It has been my experience that children who have never listened to classical music can become fascinated by this genre when they are exposed to it. They cannot have any concept of it if they have never heard classical music—only rumors that it is boring and impossible to understand. The same reasoning could be applied to various forms of visual arts, literature, and theater. If children are exposed to many forms of cultural expression, they will have a big cultural menu in their brains, and they could use that menu in many ways throughout life.

There are other ethical problems surrounding cultural activity as a tool for improving public health. Adults have different backgrounds socially and psychologically. This means that there are pronounced differences in cultural preferences. A good society should not force a specific form of cultural expression on people, some of whom may react very negatively to a given piece of music, for instance. Such exposure has been used systematically as amplification of torture, such as in Abu Ghraib, a prison camp in Iraq where Arabic prisoners were kept in American prisons and were exposed to American pop music that the prison staff knew they hated. Such problems become obvious when a work site offers cultural activities for the employees. Joint experiences can strengthen cohesiveness and stimulate creativity, resulting in reduced risk for the development of depressive feelings among employees, as we have seen in one of our epidemiological studies (Theorell & Nyberg, 2019). The solution to such problems is to respect diversity and examine ways of approaching differences in cultural preferences and needs. In this process, applied research is a necessary tool that will help us find solutions. Concerning diversity, for instance, in music preferences, no research indicates that one music genre produces better health than other genres.

D.5 Bribery and Bias in Research Publication

The classical situation in which bribery has been a problem in applied science is occupational toxicology. It is very difficult to know the extent of bribery in that field. Since that research is about possible relationships between exposure to possible toxic agents at work sites and diseases such as cancer, myocardial infarction, and stroke, there are strong financial forces that could influence communication between researchers and society. There may be financial benefits for a researcher employed by a company to minimize the importance of relationships between a toxic agent and an illness. This is, of course, against ethical rules, but unfortunately, it has occurred. There is always an employer behind a bribery of this kind, but the researcher has the responsibility for reporting.

Scientific journals have their own strict rules. The researcher who wants to publish has to honestly describe all ties to relevant parties. Such ties are then published with the article, and the reader may assess credibility: Is this group of researchers credible in this report? Most researchers are honest and follow the ethical rules, but some of them may be under pressure from large companies, which can offer large sums of money to mute the researcher group when results do not come out in the desired way, and even pay for new laboratories or employment of staff to produce desired results. Scientific journals may be under pressure not to publish inconvenient results. The general rule is that large, well-known journals with well-known editors and reviewers can resist such efforts.

Some of the largest international pharmaceutical companies run both scientific foundations that award grants to scientists who apply for them and scientific journals. Most of the scientific boards selecting research to be granted and editorial boards deciding to publish scientific reports have high ethical standards. They have indeed been able to respect the walls between the selling of pharmacological agents, vaccines, and equipment for various kinds of health care on one hand, and judgements regarding grants and publications, but there are also examples of pharmaceutical companies that have favored grants and scientific articles that lead to the recommendation of their products. The walls are sometimes thin.

Scientific journals are extremely important for the credibility in general of applied science. One problem that editors must handle is the tendency to publish reports with "positive findings," i.e., results that are in line with a popular hypothesis. Correspondingly, journals are less interested in publishing null findings that go against the popular hypothesis. This is labeled *positive publication bias*. If positive publication bias is widespread, erroneous hypotheses may spread, and this may, in the long run, contribute to diminished trust in science.

The figure below illustrates one way in which possible positive publication bias could be assessed. It shows a so-called funnel plot. The figure is based upon a meta (summarizing) study (Theorell et al., 2016) of scientifically published epidemiological studies of the relationship between working in a work situation characterized as a job with high demands and low control, amounting to a great deal of job strain. Only high-quality studies have been included, and adjustments have been made for other established risk factors. Each study has presented an odds ratio, i.e., the likelihood that a person with job strain will develop ischemic heart disease within the near future. On the y axis, the standard error of the assessed risk is represented; the smaller the standard error (which mainly means many participants in the study), the higher on the y axis. The x axis corresponds to the log (odds ratio) for each study. *Log* means that these odds ratios have been logarithmically transformed; the lower the odds ratio, the longer the distances on the x axis and vice versa. A minus sign indicates a ratio that is lower than 1.0 and vice versa. In this case, a minus sign indicates that there is a finding that runs against expectations, a higher risk of developing ischemic heart disease during follow-up among those *without* job strain. Only one study showed such a counterintuitive finding, whereas the remaining 21 studies all showed the expected direction of the relationship. However, the *funnel plot* tests whether the dots are all within the triangle. This reflects the assumption that larger studies, with more participants, have smaller statistical errors due to reduced measurement variability, whereas small studies, with fewer participants, exhibit larger errors. If there is a positive publication bias, such biased studies should be found outside the right-hand part of the lower part of the triangle since they do not conform to the statistical expectation that small studies should have a large measurement error. In this special case, the test indicates that positive publication bias is not a problem.

Figure 2 shows a funnel plot exploring possible publication bias based upon data on the possible relation of exposure to job strain to risk of developing ischemic heart disease (Theorell et al., 2016).

This method for exploring positive publication bias is not the only method for testing publication bias in surveys of many studies. There are several others.

There is also another extreme in the interpretation of scientific findings. I would label this *negative bias*, in its most extreme form, *nihilistic bias*. I have encountered this in research students when I have given lectures about rules in science. The students may, during the lecture, get the impression that no research findings are reliable. Negative bias means an attitude of severe doubt—regardless of what findings are presented, the response will always be: "No, there is variance due to other factors, some of them unknown. If you take that into account, there will be no explanatory power left." Factors labeled *confounders* could indeed give rise to spurious associations. One example is age. If both the explanatory (a) and the dependent (b) variables are more common in old than in young people, the first calculations may give the impression that there is a causal relationship between *a* and *b*. But when age has been adjusted for, it turns out that the association is totally explained by age, and *a* has no explanatory value in relation to *b* per se. In that case, age acted as a confounder, which created a spurious relationship. There are many such examples, but

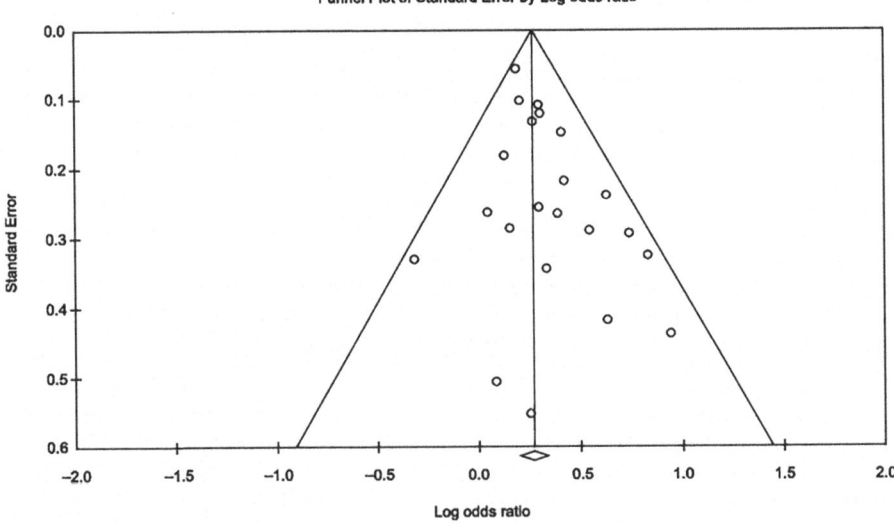

Fig. 2 Testing the likelihood of positive publication bias. Source: Theorell et al. (2016) (Reprinted from Theorell et al. (2016), Figure 3. https://doi.org/10.1093/eurpub/ckw025, licensed under the terms of the Creative Commons Attribution Non-Commercial License (http://creativecommons. org/licenses/by-nc/4.0/). Reproduced by permission of Oxford University Press on behalf of the European Public Health Association)

professional epidemiologists have mostly identified the relevant ones and taken them into account in the calculations. But one should always make sure that a professional job has been performed on these things. The next step for the nihilist is to say that unknown variables are likely to explain the finding, which is therefore declared unreliable. This is, however, not an argument that can be used, because an unknown variable, the value of which cannot be established, cannot be used to explain away an observed relationship.

In epidemiological research, a large number of potential confounders can be used. But the reader of a scientific report of that kind should also remember that the introduction of a large number of such factors *per sé* increases the insecurity in the estimates of the relationship. It is thus possible to declare a relationship unreliable by simply throwing many confounding variables into the eqs. A good judgment is thus needed for anyone reading scientific reports in judging reliability. It is important not to be too critical because that may erroneously lead to invalidation of reliable reports. Despite the obligation to critically examine how the study was performed and how the scientific rules were followed, it is also important to accept results from good studies. Nihilists can erroneously delay the acceptance of important results and prevent societal action.

References

Antonovsky, A. (1979). *Health, stress and coping.* Jossey-Bass.

Bengtsson, C., Theorell, T., Klareskog, L., & Alfredsson, L. (2009). Psychosocial stress at work and the risk of developing rheumatoid arthritis: Results from the Swedish EIRA study. *Psychotherapy and Psychosomatics, 78*(3), 193–194. https://doi.org/10.1159/000209351. Epub 2009 Mar 24.

Caselli, I., Ielmini, M., Bellini, A., Zizolfi, D., & Callegari, C. J. (2023). Efficacy of short-term psychodynamic psychotherapy (STPP) in depressive disorders: A systematic review and meta-analysis. *Journal of Affective Disorders, 325*, 169–176. https://doi.org/10.1016/j.jad.2022.12.161. Epub 2023 Jan 6. PMID: 36623570 Review.

Elander Lindberg, N. (1997). *Psychological processes in somatic disease.* Doctoral thesis, Karolinska Institutet.

Häggmark, C. (1990). Attitudes to increased involvement of relatives in the care of cancer patients. Evaluation of an activation program. *Cancer Nursing.* PMID: 2306718.

Hamrin, E., Kihlgren, M., Rinell Hermansson, A., & Östlinder, G. (Eds.). (2014). *När omvårdnad blev vetenskap (When nursing care became science).* Liber.

Henje Blom, E. C., Serlachius, E., Larsson, J.-O., Theorell, T., & Ingvar, M. (2010). Low Sense of Coherence (SOC) is a mirror of general anxiety and persistent depressive symptoms in adolescent girls - A cross-sectional study of a clinical and a non-clinical cohort. *Health and Quality of Life Outcomes, 8*, 58. https://doi.org/10.1186/1477-7525-8-58

Jacobson, B., Nyberg, K., Grönbladh, L., Eklund, G., Bygdeman, M., & Rydberg, U. (1990). Opiate addiction in adult offspring through possible imprinting after obstetric treatment. *BMJ, 301*(6760), 1067–1070. https://doi.org/10.1136/bmj.301.6760.1067

Jeong, H. J., Durham, E. L., Moore, T. M., Dupont, R. M., McDowell, M., Cardenas-Iniguez, C., Micciche, E. T., Berman, M. G., Lahey, B. B., & Kaczkurkin, A. N. (2021). The association between latent trauma and brain structure in children. *Translational Psychiatry, 11*(1), 240. https://doi.org/10.1038/s41398-021-01357-z

Johansson Palmqvist, Å., Borgström, D., & Björkstén, U. VA-barometern 2024/2025 – VA-rapport. isbn 978-91-89039-27-82024 :4 Vetenskap och Allmänhet.

Josefsson, D. (2013). *Mannen som slutade ljuga (The man who stopped lying)*. Lind & Co Falun.

Meslé, M. M. I., et al. (2024 Sep). Estimated number of lives directly saved by COVID-19 vaccination programmes in the WHO European Region from December, 2020, to March, 2023: A retrospective surveillance study. *Respiratory Medicine, 12*(9), 714–727. https://doi.org/10.1016/S2213-2600(24)00179-6

Nilsson, B., Holmgren, L., Stegmayr, B., & Westman, G. (2003). Sense of coherence--stability over time and relation to health, disease, and psychosocial changes in a general population: A longitudinal study. *Scandinavian Journal of Public Health, 31*(4), 297–304. https://doi.org/10.1080/14034940210164920

Öst, L. G., Enebrink, P., Finnes, A., Ghaderi, A., Havnen, A., Kvale, G., Salomonsson, S., & Wergeland, G. J. (2023). Cognitive behavior therapy for adult depressive disorders in routine clinical care: A systematic review and meta-analysis. *Journal of Affective Disorders, 331*, 322–333. https://doi.org/10.1016/j.jad.2023.03.002. Epub 2023 Mar 8. PMID: 36894029 Review.

Råstam, H. (2017). *Fallet Thomas Quick: att skapa en seriemördare (Thomas Quick: To create a mass murderer)*. Ordfront. 9789174411515.

Szyf, M. (2012). Mind-body interrelationship in DNA methylation. *Chemical Immunology and Allergy, 90*, 85–99.

Theorell, T. (2016). Arts, health and job stress. In *Developing leadership and employee health through the arts*. Springer. https://doi.org/10.1007/987-3-319-41969-5_1

Theorell, T., & Nyberg, A. (2019). Cultural activity at work: reciprocal associations with depressive symptoms in employees. *International Archives of Occupational and Environmental Health, 92*(8), 1131–1137. https://doi.org/10.1007/s00420-019-01452-1. Epub 2019 Jun 11.

Theorell, T., Häggmark, C., & Eneroth, P. (1987). Psycho-endocrinological reactions in female relatives of cancer patients. Effects of an activation programme. *Acta Oncologica, 26*(6), 419–424. https://doi.org/10.3109/02841868709113710

Theorell, T., Jood, K., Järvholm, L. S., Vingård, E., Perk, J., Östergren, P. O., & Hall, C. (2016). A systematic review of studies in the contributions of the work environment to ischaemic heart disease development. *European Journal of Public Health, 26*(3), 470–477. https://doi.org/10.1093/eurpub/ckw025. Epub 2016 Mar 31.

Wahlberg, V. (1982). Reconsideration of Credé prophylaxis. A study of maternity and neonatal care. *Acta Paediatrica Scandinavica. Supplement, 295*, 1–73.

Examples of Situations in Which Applied Science Should Have Been Used More

In order to make the questions regarding the role society gives to applied science more concrete, we need examples that can stimulate discussions in a teaching situation.

I will first present a question, and then for each of them, a list of conditions that should be discussed before a reasonable decision can be made regarding interpretation.

1. **An advertisement states that treatment with a nasal spray of oxytocin twice daily for two months will make your teenager less shy. According to the advertisement, this has been supported by research performed in a famous university**

   Is there previously published research which could make it likely that it is possible that oxytocin could cure shyness? Yes—this is not completely out of the blue—because there is research published in reliable scientific journals showing that oxytocin has a role in *togetherness* or *attachment* situations—for instance, when people are singing together, when skin is touched, or otherwise when conditions allow a safe social connection. This information is available in scientific databases. However, that does not prove that external input of oxytocin on a daily basis would cure shyness. When hormones are added to the body artificially, there are often adaptive processes that change the effects after some time, and we do not know what the long-term effects of nasally added oxytocin might be in the long run. Before we have such reliable information, we should hesitate to take this advertisement seriously. There is also an ongoing scientific debate about whether nasal oxytocin reaches the brain or not. We should ideally understand how a possible oxytocin effect arises. Maybe the nasal oxytocin has peripheral effects that affect the brain secondarily. If so, we should perhaps instead look for the real agent if oxytocin is only indirectly involved. Finally, is shyness in a teenager necessarily a bad thing? Maybe shyness in a developmental

T. Theorell, *Underuse of Applied Science in Changing Societies*, SpringerBriefs in Public Health, https://doi.org/10.1007/978-3-031-96391-9_6

stage is useful? This discussion is at a very early stage, and the participants in the discussion can conduct research in scientific databases.

2. **A politician is trying to convince his/her potential electors that privately administered primary health care centers are much more effective than primary health care centers administered by counties or municipalities.**

Is there any scientific support for such a statement? Yes, on a superficial level, some studies present such results. However, one should read those studies carefully. First, in some of the comparisons of primary care in the two main groups—private and public centers—the comparison is unfair because the private centers can select their patients, whereas the public centers are forced to serve all patients. This varies greatly between countries and between counties, but in general, this is the case. This means that private centers can select younger patients with easy-to-treat conditions and dismiss the others. Consequently, the public health care centers will have a larger remaining proportion of patients with high age, multi-morbidity, and abuse of drugs and alcohol than the private centers. This means that each patient consultation takes a longer time in the public centers. To some extent, laws can compensate for some of this, but experience from our country has shown that the disadvantage for the public centers is considerable. If comparisons are made without adjustment for these disadvantages, one may erroneously get the impression that public care is less efficient *per sé* than private care. In health care fully financed by taxes, there is a limited monetary space for establishing private care centers, and during many years of unregulated new establishment of such centers the consequence has been that low-income areas with a poor public health status sometimes have seen their only health care center close down forcing people to travel long distances for medical consultations and treatments. On the other hand, those living in high-income areas will see the establishment of too many private health care centers consuming money from the limited financial funds allocated to the area, which creates difficulties for those centers that must treat everybody. One other consequence is that it is impossible to establish an area-based prevention plan. When there is no responsibility for a defined area and inhabitants are scattered across a large area unrelated to the center's geographical position, it is not possible to establish effective prevention in the area.

On the one hand, most reports that paint a rosy picture of private care should be read critically. On the other hand, independence for a health care center is indeed beneficial from many points of view. It may be easier to establish a good work environment in private care, which may have a simpler work organization, for instance. Thus, the solutions will have to take into consideration several complicated arguments, and the truth is not simple. What weight shall I, as a citizen, give to different arguments? A private health care center may be good for me, personally, but it is also valuable to me that citizens with small financial resources have good health care. Applied science has tools for stimulating reasonable arguments from different points of view, and it is accordingly a pity that politicians do not allow the scientific arguments to weigh heavily in political discussions. Ideological arguments frequently dominate in the final decisions. If basic health care needs are not met for large groups of citizens, we have a bad society, and that will affect everybody, also those with good resources.

3. **Local politicians in a city want to retain a small airport located in the city itself (for example, Bromma in Stockholm).**

    How can results from applied science help the decision process?

    The airport is located within a heavily populated area—Stockholm. It has been shown in epidemiological studies that airport noise may raise morning cortisol concentration in women living close to airports (Selander et al., 2009). In addition, studies have also shown effects on blood pressure and the incidence of myocardial infarction in people living close to airports. Accordingly, there are documented adverse health effects that should be taken into account. As we read in newspapers, there have also been disasters with airplane crashes upon take-off or landing, causing deaths, which have occurred twice in the history of this airport. The risks of such adverse consequences should be evaluated against possible benefits. In my country, politicians do take the adverse consequences into account, but despite this, the decision to close this airport near Stockholm has been delayed for several decades (1958–2025). It has been argued that the proximity of the airport to central Stockholm is a great advantage for business in Stockholm. These kinds of comparisons between risks and benefits in different spheres of societal activity are particularly difficult, but in this case, applied health science has not played the important role that could be expected in decision-making. Other arguments that have not been seriously discussed are related to carbon dioxide dissemination concerning air traffic. Such discussions are highly complex, since one has to take into consideration carbon dioxide dissemination not only from the airplanes but also from car driving to and from the airport. One also has to perform calculations of the effects of changes arising due to the fact that car travelers may have to drive their cars for longer distances if the air traffic is moved outside the city. The balance between public transportation (buses and trains) and private car driving also has to be taken into account, as well as the extent to which cars are electrified, and so on. Admittedly, the decision process is a difficult one, but various fields of applied science should be used before decisions are taken.

4. **The long process of admitting the link between tobacco smoking and lung cancer is interesting** *because it shows the strong influence that industry may have on society's interpretation of results coming from applied science.*

    As I mentioned in the introduction, my father, who was a typical representative of basic scientists (biochemists) in the 1940s to the 1980s ("When you need statistics for proving something it is not science anymore"), was for a long time not willing to accept that there could be a link between tobacco smoking and lung cancer. He even mocked evidence from epidemiological research, being himself an enthusiastic tobacco smoker and friend of the director of the Swedish monopoly of the cigarette industry. He even showed his contempt by smoking at public events. He did, however, change his mind in the late 1970s.

    Proctor (2012) has described this long process in the following summary:

Lung cancer was once a very rare disease, so rare that doctors took special notice when confronted with a case, thinking it a once-in-a-lifetime oddity. Mechanization and mass marketing towards the end of the nineteenth century popularized the cigarette habit, however, causing a global lung cancer epidemic. Cigarettes were recognized as the cause of the epidemic in the 1940s and 1950s, with the confluence of studies from epidemiology, animal experiments, cellular pathology and chemical analytics. Cigarette manufacturers disputed this evidence as part of an orchestrated conspiracy to salvage cigarette sales. Propagandizing the public proved successful, judging from secret tobacco industry measurements of the impact of denialist propaganda. As late as 1960 only one-third of all US doctors believed that the case against cigarettes had been established. Cigarettes cause about 1.5 million deaths per year.

It has been estimated that cigarette makers make about a penny in profit for every cigarette sold, which means that the value of a life to a cigarette maker is about 10,000 U.S. dollars.

Although the tobacco industry managed to slow down the process, there is today a general awareness of the harmful effects of tobacco smoking, and the prevalence of smoking has decreased dramatically in many countries.

5. **Factories Polluting Japanese Water with Serious Consequences**

The two famous Japanese environmental disasters, Itai-itai (Mehdikhan-mahaleh & Tabatabaei-Malazy, 2024) and Minamata (Harada, 1995), illustrate how toxic industries polluting water in their neighborhoods can delay relevant action for decades despite ample evidence from applied science that their leakage of poison caused severe illness and increased local mortality. In the older example, Minamata, it was mercury causing the problem, whereas in the newer example, cadmium poisoning was the culprit. The Minamata disease was due to the wastewater, with methyl mercury polluting the Minamata Bay, and when people ate marine products from the Bay, they developed symptoms. The connection was discovered by scientists as early as 1956, but it was not until 1968 that the pollution was forced to stop. The victims had neurological symptoms, and children born to mothers with a high content of methyl mercury had severe congenital brain disorders. Itai-itai arose during and after World War II in the production of batteries, which gave rise to cadmium compounds polluting the Jinzu River bay. Women, especially, were affected by the disease, which resulted in severe symptoms, in particular pain, in the bones. The disease and its etiology were described in 1955, and in 1968, the government admitted the connection officially. The take-home message from both these examples was that both those responsible for industry and, to some extent, local administrators and politicians delayed effective action. The industry did not want their activity hindered, and the local administrators and politicians wanted to keep jobs in the region. In both cases, the employers were among the few employers in the region, and they had large numbers of employees.

6. **Psychosocial Work Environment**

I have discussed in some detail earlier about how a poor psychosocial work environment can give rise to large-scale health problems in the working population as well as considerable loss of productivity. Calculations have shown that substantial savings could be made both for companies and society if psychosocial risk factors at work could be reduced (McDaid et al., 2019; OECD, 2014; Hassard et al., 2017). If employers become more aware of all possible sources of financial losses due to a poor psychosocial work environment, this could improve active participation. It is already true that many employers and managers rate quality-of-life factors at work as more important in the competition than financial arguments.

But there are many companies that do not take the work environment messages seriously and do not realize the potential financial gains that could be obtained with improved management.

There is, for instance, a growing literature exploring whether cultural activity organized for employees can decrease the risk of worsening depressive states. Our example in our research (Theorell & Nyberg, 2019) was based upon a large longitudinal study of Swedish employees in which the degree of depression related to aspects of the work environment, including cultural activities in the workplace, was assessed before it, and then again two years later. The findings showed that employees who reported that their workplace organized cultural activities for the employees had a lower risk of developing depression after two years than other participants. But it was also shown that subjects who were depressed at the start participated less in the cultural activities than others, which is a pity, since they would have benefited from participation in those activities more than other employees.

A frequently reported reason for low participation in discussions about work environment interventions among managers is that they may be afraid of becoming openly criticized in group meetings with staff. Employees may also fear such situations. When several parts are involved, open confrontations may be feared by all. Avoidance may be the result. Antagonists on both sides may accordingly actively avoid constructive dialogue. There are solutions to such avoidance problems, however.

7. Low-Frequency Noise from Wind Turbines and Health Effects

Since wind turbines seem to offer one possible solution to some of the growing energy problems in the world, responsible societies mustn't rush through the building of enormous parks of wind turbines before we know how to protect ourselves against possible adverse health effects. Such effects have indeed been shown in epidemiological studies. For instance, Poulsen et al. (2019) showed in Denmark in a large epidemiological study that among elderly living close to wind turbines with a high level of low-frequency noise, the consumption of anti-depressive medication was significantly elevated. Similar findings were made for sleep medication, although these results were only borderline significant. Chiu et al. (2021) used a more objective outcome: heart rate variability. They could show that components of heart rate variability that are related to the activity in the parasympathetic system (antistress) diminished significantly among subjects living close to wind turbines when the intensity of low-frequency noise was high outdoors. If such effects are widespread, they may affect blood pressure levels and the risk of heart disease among people. The results furthermore seemed to indicate that the low-frequency noise indoors in concrete houses was lower than in other kinds of houses close to wind turbines. The authors concluded that there should be regulations for house building in proximity to wind turbines. McCunney et al. (2014), in a review of published research, concluded that some of the reported health effects could be "annoyance" effects, which should be taken seriously—as we know from psychophysiological research, long-lasting exposure to annoyance can cause permanent physiological disturbance. Although the effects are relatively small, they are important on a population level since large numbers of people are potentially affected. The wind turbines are getting progressively bigger, and they produce very low-frequency noise, the effects of which are unknown. And outdoor conditions make a substantial difference. With frequency as low as 1 Hz in combination with strong winds and low temperature, the biological effects can be strong (Keith et al., 2018). In addition, there are discussions regarding possible effects on cattle, poultry, as well as wild animals such as prairie chickens and dolphins. Although this is an ongoing scientific discussion, it is important that society pays active attention to and supports such research so that we can protect both humans and nature effectively in the future. This is already affecting large numbers of people and animals in the world and is likely to cause extensive effects on public health. There is a tendency among politicians to actively disregard research on the adverse effects of wind turbines.

8. **The Climate Question**

Perhaps the most important scientific question of our time is how we can stop the ongoing, increasingly dramatic climate change. I am not going to describe the complicated basic science process underlying the conclusions that scientists have arrived at. For decades, there were deep conflicts between different groups of scientists, but today there is an almost unified conclusion among earth scientists: The continuation on the present scale of carbon dioxide pollution in the atmosphere will result in a dramatic deterioration of the Earths climate. We also know that there will be more floods in highly populated areas as well as more hurricanes of hitherto unknown intensity, and an increasing number of wildfires in wooded areas.

A big surprise for me is that this new climatological scientific knowledge has not been accepted by everybody, and, even more surprisingly, a decrease in the percentage of people considering climate change to be a threat was observed in several areas of the world (Capstick et al., 2014). Between 2007–2008 and 2010, there was a 10% decrease in the United States and Western Europe and a 7% decrease in Eastern and Southern Europe. One reason that has been proposed for this counterintuitive trend in these populations is that the worldwide financial crisis in 2008 had a major effect, and that this may have decreased the focus on the climate crisis. In other countries, the trends were in the opposite direction, a 12—24% increase in people considering climate change to be a threat (Mongolia, Philippines, Ecuador, Uganda, and Morocco). This may be an illustration of the difficulties we face when we try to solve a serious worldwide problem, the solution of which requires deep cuts and major changes in people's way of living their lives. When a major financial crisis occurs in some countries, many citizens may consider other societal problems (such as a financial crisis) more important than climate change.

Competing priorities may explain why politicians do not focus on the climate problem, although this is potentially of such enormous significance to all of us. Another reason may be the short cycles in politics. In many countries, politicians are elected for four-year periods, and they want to be reelected. This means that questions that have to be solved by means of processes taking many years and the results of which are not foreseeable within a short time period will be under-prioritized. Unfortunately, the politicians who favor short-term solutions may rapidly gain popularity. They may even amplify their popularity by accusing the scientists of faking their data, and hence, diminish trust in applied science. One solution to such problems could be longer cycles for political decisions regarding far-reaching, important questions that are of particular importance for coming generations. Another point should be the development of increased knowledge in the population regarding how scientific knowledge is being built. Such changes require careful planning and devotion of considerable amounts of time.

Regarding climate change, it is necessary to invent adapted proposals for change. It has been pointed out, in Sweden for instance, that people living in the countryside may be less willing to make fundamental changes in their ways of living. But this is not due to unwillingness in general to accept the importance of climate change; it is rather related to their specific life habits (Pelling, 2024). For instance, those who live far outside cities depend heavily on the use of cars. They have less money than those living in the cities, and therefore, they cannot afford to buy electric cars. At the same time, public transportation facilities have been shrinking—fewer train connections reduce the possibility of getting public transportation; in some cases, pharmacies and health care centers have closed, as well as primary and secondary schools. All of this results in more long-distance private transportation with carbon dioxide pollution. If politicians want to take serious steps to reduce carbon dioxide pollution, they will have to incorporate political actions that specifically address different kinds of lifestyles.

References

Capstick, S., Whitmarsh, L., Poortinga, W., Pidgeon, N., & Upham, P. (2014). International trends in public perceptions of climate change over the past quarter century. *WIREs Climate Change.* https://doi.org/10.1002/wcc.321

Chiu, C.-H., Lung, S.-C. C., Chen, N., & Tsou, M.-C. M. (2021). Effects of low-frequency noise from wind turbines on heart rate variability in healthy individuals. *Scientific Reports, 11,* 17817.

Harada, M. (1995). Minamata disease: Methylmercury poisoning in Japan caused by environmental pollution. *Critical Reviews in Toxicology, 25*(1), 1–24. https://doi.org/10.3109/10408449509089885

Hassard, J., Teoh, K. R. H., Visockaite, G., Dewe, P., & Cox, T. (2017). The cost of work-related stress to society: A systematic review. *Journal of Occupational Health Psychology.*

Keith, S. E., Daigle, G. A., & Stinson, M. R. (2018). Wind turbine low frequency and infrasound propagation and sound pressure level calculations at dwellings. *Journal of the Acoustical Society of America, 144,* 981–996. https://doi.org/10.1121/1.5051331

McCunney, R. J., Mundt, K. A., Colby, W. D., Dobie, R., Kaliski, K., & Blais, M. J. (2014). Wind turbines and health: A critical review of the scientific literature. *Occupational and Environmental Medicine, 56*(11), e108-30. https://doi.org/10.1097/JOM.0000000000000313. PMID: 25376420 Review.

McDaid, D., Park, A., & Wahlbeck, K. (2019). The economic case for the prevention of mental illness. *Annual Review of Public Health, 40,* 373–389.

Mehdikhanmahaleh, M. M., & Tabatabaei-Malazy, M. (2024). *Itai itai disease Encyclopedia of toxicology* (Vol. 5, 4th ed., pp. 725–729). https://doi.org/10.1016/B978-0-12-824315-2.00924-6

OECD. (2014). *Making mental health count: The social and economic costs of neglecting mental health care. OECD health policy studies.* OECD.

Pelling, L. (2024, July 8). *Climate capabilities: Realising the green transition.* Social Europe.

Poulsen, A. H., Raaschou-Nielsen, O., Peña, A., Hahmann, A. N., Nordsborg, R. B., Ketzel, M., Brandt, J., & Sørensen, M. (2019). Impact of Long-term exposure to wind turbine noise on redemption of sleep medication and antidepressants: A Nationwide Cohort Study. *Environmental Health Perspectives, 127*(3), 37005. https://doi.org/10.1289/EHP3909

Proctor, R. N. (2012). The history of the discovery of the cigarette-lung cancer link – Evidentiary traditions, corporate denial, global toll. *Tobacco Control, 21*(2), 87–91. https://doi.org/10.1136/tobaccocontrol-2011-050338

Selander, J., Bluhm, G., Theorell, T., Pershagen, G., Babisch, W., Seiffert, I., Houthuijs, D., Breugelmans, O., Vigna-Taglianti, F., Antoniotti, M. C., Velonakis, E., Davou, E., Dudley, M. L., Järup, L., & HYENA Consortium. (2009). Saliva cortisol and exposure to aircraft noise in six European countries. *Environmental Health Perspectives, 117*(11), 1713–1717. https://doi.org/10.1289/ehp.0900933. Epub 2009 Jul 20. PMID: 20049122.

Theorell, T., & Nyberg, A. (2019). Cultural activity at work: Reciprocal associations with depressive symptoms in employees. *International Archives of Occupational and Environmental Health, 92*(8), 1131–1137. https://doi.org/10.1007/s00420-019-01452-1. Epub 2019 Jun 11.

Solutions

F1. How to Improve the Situation?

In discussing what we can do to improve the position for applied research in society, I shall move from the inside outwards. This means that I start with the researchers themselves.

The credibility and the societal position of applied science depend largely on the researchers´ ability to maintain a high ethical standard. The most obvious examples of faked results or grossly exaggerated positive findings (such as the Macchiarini example mentioned in the chapter "How Does Applied Science Operate?" (p. XX) are not common, but I have also mentioned that there are twilight zones in scientific production.

The *mass significance* problem occurs in studies with many possible explanatory variables. Conducting multiple statistical tests at a 5% significance level heightens the risk of falsely accepting a random result as significant. A 5% limit for acceptance means that if one tests a relationship over and over again, a 5% significance requirement for accepting the relationship as *statistically significant* is that one has to make the test more than twenty times to find a *false* result that is in reality only a chance finding. But if two tests are done at the same time using the same statistical 5% requirement, the likelihood doubles that one of them could seem statistically significant, simply because the number of tests has increased. Common procedures for solving this problem are:

(a) Raise the demand for statistical significance, for example, to 1 in 100
(b) Multiply the significance level 0.04 (in my example) by the number of tests. According to this latter reasoning, the *real* significance level should be 0.08 (two tests multiplied by 0.04), which is not significant if we use <0.05 as our limit. Both of those approaches are problematic, mainly because the risk increases that we reject a relationship as true, although it could be true. However, in this situation, the researchers should disclose how many tests were made.

T. Theorell, *Underuse of Applied Science in Changing Societies*, SpringerBriefs in Public Health, https://doi.org/10.1007/978-3-031-96391-9_7

This makes it possible for the receiver of the report to accept or reject the finding. Accordingly, hiding the fact that many tests were performed that were not reported is in the ethical dark zone. The researchers could also examine whether the finding is biologically plausible or plausible for other reasons, and in that way throw light on the degree of credibility. This could be useful, but it could also be ethically dangerous. How does one define plausibility? As always, the real issue is honesty. If researchers are honest and openly discuss the pros and cons when they describe their findings, they leave it to other researchers to accept or reject their interpretations. If society can see that the researchers do indeed follow their own rules, it increases the science's credibility among lay people. Indeed, some researchers work tirelessly on improving researcher honesty by giving courses and writing articles and textbooks about it.

There is growing concern among scientists that liberal application of and interpretation of statistical analyses may lead to spurious diversity. Gould et al. (2025) published two examples from an unpublished study in which a large number of researchers were asked to perform statistical analyses on the same dataset and interpret them. They found that these researchers found widely differing results, even though they were working with the same data set. This emphasizes the importance of adherence to rigid rules for statistical interpretation.

An important group in the communication between researchers and society is the journalists. Both journalists and researchers have important responsibilities. The first rule for researchers and journalists is to abstain from communicating results to society before they have been discussed and confirmed by the research community. This could either mean that the results have been described in a report that has been accepted for publication in a respected journal (thus, not a "predator" according to Beall's list; see above) or at least been discussed in a congress in which knowledgeable scholars have been present. It often happens that scientific discussion leads to changes in the interpretation of the results, and hence, premature promulgation of findings could hurt the credibility of the researchers. Journalists, on the other hand, have the responsibility to pose critical questions to the researcher and to describe weaknesses as well as strengths in the resulting articles. Ideally, journalists writing about research results should be aware of scientific rules for publication, and they should also resist pressure from influential groups to publish biased results to lay people.

Scientific journals and their editors should also resist pressure from the outside. In general, they are obliged to avoid "publication bias" (see the Chapter "Communication With Society"; [p. XX]), both in the form of willingness to please groups with financial power, and in general, favoring positive findings at the expense of negative ones, since the positive findings may attract a bigger readership and in some circumstances, please politicians. This requires a systematic effort, and all editors, not only those in large, established, top-ranked journals, must be taught how to expedite such efforts.

The conclusion is that researchers, editors of scientific journals, journalists describing scientific results for lay people, and lay people themselves must learn more about how science works. Everyone must know the basic rules governing how science works. This should start at school. Ideally, a new subject should be introduced—*scientific interpretation knowledge*. I do not know which major subject it would be included in—Philosophy, Mathematics, or Civics. Perhaps it should be part of all these subjects. Everyone in society should know how science works so that it is not a myopic activity performed by scientists who lack knowledge about the real world. In addition, everyone should know that all kinds of applied sciences try to describe the real world as correctly as possible, and that rules are followed regarding data collection and computation of statistical relationships. Everyone should also know that intense discussions between scientists are normal before a consensus has been obtained. Scientists should also be better prepared for honest discussions with lay people regarding such things as representativeness of participants in a research project, choice of statistics, and precision of examination methods.

F2. Science and Politics

When the politicians in power are not interested in listening to science, viewing it as disturbing noise that hinders their plans, it is difficult to make science important in society. A somewhat paranoid interpretation of the reasons for reduced resources to society's support of applied science (for instance, research about material and psychosocial resources and needs in different parts of society) is that some groups of politicians actively do not want us all to know about injustice in society. A major obstacle to the wise utilization of scientific knowledge is short election periods. In my country, politicians are elected for four years. Election periods vary between countries, but a general problem is that the cycles are short. If the politicians´ only egocentric concern is to be reelected, it is very hard to defend long-term goals supported by scientific arguments. This becomes particularly problematic when very long cycles must be considered, such as climate change, especially if a decrease in long-term predicted adverse consequences causes demands for societal and individual changes that are unpopular. However, it could be argued that when knowledge about how applied science functions becomes more widespread, even the most egoistic politicians will have to listen to scientifically based arguments, because they increasingly hear those kinds of discussions and because people who elect them know what applied science is about and what it could be used for. This may be a very extended process. However, there are signs that some parts of a scientific attitude to news may already be underway in modern schools. Workshops are organized for teachers (Powell & Hood, 2023). *Source critique* is being taught in secondary schools in many countries, and there are signs that younger generations are more aware of the importance of source awareness than older ones. Textbooks are also available (Rosenqvist & Ekecrantz, 2023).

In an ideal world, the principles of scientific thinking should be part of societal thinking. How can risks and benefits be calculated or expressed in objective terms?

I have already mentioned the theatrical trilogy *The Oresteia* by Aeschylus (see Chapter "Communication with Society," [p. XX]). It had its first performance in 458 BC. Aeschylus wrote this play for the Athenians because he wanted to teach civilized ways of solving conflicts. The theatrical stage was the arena for such teaching. In his time, murders and violence were the most common methods for solving conflicts. If Aeschylus had lived today, he might have proposed the use of applied science for solving conflicts. Today, we have applied science, but we do not use it as frequently as we should.

References

Gould, E., Fraser, H. S., Parker, T. H., et al. (2025). Same data, different analysis: Variation in effect sizes due to analytical decisions in ecology and evolutionary biology. *BMC Biology, 23*(1), 35. https://doi.org/10.1186/s12915-024-02101-x

Powell, E., & Hood, S. (2023). Helping students to learn how to critically evaluate a source: How effective are the tools we use? *Journal of Learning Development in Higher Education, 29.* https://doi.org/10.47408/jldhe.vi29.990

Rosenqvist, A., & Ekecrantz, S. (2023). *Source criticism on the schedule: Teaching critical thinking. Springer texts in education* (1st ed.). Springer.

Conclusions

This book has provided an overview of the conditions necessary for society to regain its trust in applied science. I started with a general discussion regarding the difference between basic and applied science. For several reasons, applied science has a weaker position in society than basic science. This is unfair because applied science can help society develop balanced and wise decisions to solve difficult problems. It could serve as a judge and as a professional aid in problem-solving.

Most of the examples related to research that I have been involved in myself are in one country—Sweden. But there is reason to believe that problems are very similar in other parts of the world, and related to other topics in applied science, although my own experiences have been confined to psychosomatic medicine, social medicine, and fine arts in the field of health work.

I have described situations in which applied science has gone wrong, but also successful international enterprises in which large numbers of participants contributed data, and researchers in many countries collaborated successfully in a joint project. I have also described how researchers, as well as the authors and journalists who publish research results, can create rules against faking, distorting, biasing, and amplifying doubtful data.

In addition, I have tried to discuss how researchers are recruited, and how the nature of research has changed over the decades encompassing my professional research adventure.

One of the most important tasks in the near future will be to increase general knowledge of how applied research works. Such education should start, primarily, in regular schools, but also take place in society at large.

T. Theorell, *Underuse of Applied Science in Changing Societies*, SpringerBriefs in Public Health, https://doi.org/10.1007/978-3-031-96391-9_8

Index

© The Author(s), under exclusive license to Springer Nature
Switzerland AG 2025
T. Theorell, *Underuse of Applied Science in Changing Societies*, SpringerBriefs
in Public Health, https://doi.org/10.1007/978-3-031-96391-9

The manufacturer's authorised representative in the EU is Springer
Nature Customer Service Centre GmbH, Europaplatz 3, 69115 Heidelberg,
Germany. If you have any concerns regarding our products, please
contact ProductSafety@springernature.com

Printed and bound by CPI Group (UK) Ltd, Croydon, CR0 4YY
28/04/2026
02098544-0001